Regarding the Death of My Father

Lawrence Krubner

Copyright © 2020 Lawrence Krubner
Cover photo by Ralph Krubner
Cover design by Leah McCloskey
Book design by Leah McCloskey
ISBN 9780998997643
10 9 8 7 6 5 4 3 2 1

Regarding the Death of My Father

Lawrence Krubner

Introduction

Some teenagers keep journals, but I couldn't. I needed an audience, even if that audience was just a single person.

When I was twelve years old, I went to a summer camp and made many friends. When we'd all returned to our home towns and started school again, we kept in touch by mail. (This was pre-Internet and before email was as common as it is now.) By the time I was in my late teens, I had a pretty well-established habit of understanding my life through writing letters. When my family went skiing, or the time we were in a car accident, or the time my pet gerbil escaped and ran around the house for three days before we found it – every event was fodder for letters I'd write to friends, and writing the letters helped me better understand how I felt about each event.

Self-expression in adulthood and in my career were shaped by this. When I was on staff at companies such as Shanken Publications or Teem Ventures, I leaned on email much more than other managers—until I learned that most people hated email and preferred direct verbal communication, at which point I had to adjust my style.

Given this history you can imagine that when faced with the death of my father I wrote a great deal of email to my friends. For me, it was the most natural way to process the overwhelming sorrow I felt.

My father was a photographer, and he taught me photography. Some of his ideas about what made an image powerful shaped my ideas about great writing. Above all, he emphasized seeing and documenting the details. He captured thousands of close-ups of butterflies, beetles, and flowers, before auto-focus macro lenses made this less of a challenge.

"What are the details?" he'd ask, and "Are they in focus?" My father would push me to find the essential component that invites an outsider into the scene. I translated his ideas on photography to the task of writing, with dialogue serving as my favorite method for bringing the specifics into focus. When all else fails, if I can simply write down what people said, I feel that I've captured the fulcrum on which a scene pivots. For that reason, when things at the hospital got bad for my father, I started writing down everything I said, or my father said, or the nurses said, or the doctors said.

I found a number of these emails in my archive (I've saved all of my email since 1996), describing in detail the lead-up of my father's death in 2007. In Part I, I share with you exactly how emotionally wrenching it was to say goodbye to him.

The first few emails you'll read are merely informational. I wrote them when I still thought my father might live for several more years. Later, when I realized he would soon die, I switched to a different style. I wanted very much to communicate to my friends how important my father was to me. So I started writing of incidents from my childhood, moments of joy we had shared. I also wrote of the confusion I began experiencing in dealing with the medical system responsible for his care. As both of my parents had enjoyed excellent health up to this point, they had very little experience with this aspect of life. The paradox of good health and long life is that when old age finally appears, it can feel like an ambush, catching us unawares.

Later, when my mom became seriously ill with pneumonia in 2019, I had to confront the medical bureaucracy again, and endure her own resistance to accepting help from me and from health care professionals. I found myself writing emails again. This comprises Part II.

Part III contains my contemplations regarding the health care system in the United States as it currently stands. Death must eventually come for everyone we love: many families face their greatest crisis when they're at their weakest. I offer some suggestions about how things should change to make such awful transitions a bit easier on the families.

Prologue

On the events that occurred during the year leading up to my father's death:

December 2006. My girlfriend Laura and I were living in Charlottesville, Virginia. We were business partners, running a successful web-design firm. My mother and father came to visit, and they stayed at the Omni Hotel on the Downtown Mall. We had a very good time together, though my father seemed somewhat subdued. Typically he had stories to share, but here he surprised me with his quiet demeanor. I saw him nervously tapping his fingers at one point and I was astonished. I'd never seen him do that before, and he seemed late in age—he was seventy-eight—to pick up such a habit.

March 2007. Laura and I visited my parents for a week at their home in Jackson, New Jersey. We went for some long walks in the park and had some good conversations about the creative needs of our clients. My parents seemed eager to hear how well things were going for me and Laura. However, twice during the week, my parents slipped away to some mysterious meeting which they wouldn't tell us about. I thought perhaps they were talking with bankers about refinancing their house, but I was somewhat on edge. Part of me was aware that they would be only secretive about a health matter.

Late March 2007. A week after Laura and I went back to Virginia, my father called me and let me know that he'd been diagnosed with cancer of the esophagus. My father had never smoked and had no confirmed risk factors, but he had often had trouble swallowing, which was attributed to a hiatal hernia. A different couple might have, many decades earlier, gone for surgery to get the problem fixed — but my parents had gone through life with the feeling that any medical intervention carried its own set of risks, so if a problem was minor, it did not necessarily warrant medical attention.

He admitted that his problem swallowing had suddenly started to get worse in 2006, and at some point he'd begun to suspect that he was dealing with a new problem.

When my father called me, I knew nothing about cancer of the esophagus. I didn't know the chances of survival were very poor. I was too frightened to research the issue, so I accepted my parents' assurances that my father would do some radiation therapy and chemo, and then everything would be fine. They both suggested that Laura and I should concentrate our energy on building our business and not worry. Laura and I would soon seal a deal on our biggest contract ever, so it was tempting to stay focused on work. All the same, we decided we would go north again in May to visit.

May 2007. When we arrived, my father was suffering through the worst of the radiation. I cannot easily describe how terrible it was for me to see him so weak. Still, it was Laura's birthday, and we all wanted to celebrate. Laura was a photographer, just like my father, so we went to the International Center of Photography in New York City. They had an exhibit of Henri Cartier-Bresson, a favorite of Laura's and my father. At no point in my life had I ever seen my father behave in an irritable manner, but now he was easily agitated on this day trip and lost his temper several times. It was a shock to see his personality shift, and it served as a clue about how much pain he was in. After we got home, Laura warned me that I should prepare for the worst.

August 2007. I visited Jackson alone. My father was done with his course of radiation and had regained his strength. The lump in his esophagus was gone and he was able to eat freely. We went out for long walks, we went to bookstores, and we went down to the ocean. I was elated that he'd bounced back to such an extent. At that time, I had no idea what a roller coaster cancer could be. For one month to be terrible and another month surprisingly good is, apparently, a normal part of the illness.

November 2007. My mother called me to let me know that my father had fallen down. The cancer had spread to his spine. Then she gave the phone to my father. My father warned me that he would probably never stand up again. This was a very difficult thing for me to hear, and I'm sure it was an extraordinarily difficult thing for him to say. He'd been moved to a medical rehabilitation clinic where he would receive more radiation and physical therapy. Still, he warned me, there was very little hope for him. I found that I had difficulty breathing as I tried to absorb this and process it as the truth. I told him that I would see him soon.

Early December 2007. I headed north again to New Jersey with the thought that I would stay a few weeks with my parents. I was hoping my father might live another year or at least a few more months, but just in case his time was short, I planned to spend as much time as possible with him.

Part I

Regarding My Father's Illness

Subject: *chemo is awful*
Date: *December 8, 2007*

Dear Misty,

I spent a few more hours hanging out with my dad today. It is a little strange, right now. My mom is acting as if my dad is recovering from a physical injury, like a broken leg, and so she seems to think it's only a matter of time before Dad is all better. I guess that is denial at work.

When I came into the rehab center today, my mom and dad were sitting at a table in the community room. Each of them was reading a detective novel. They've both gotten very into detective novels in recent years. I can remember a year ago, the last time they visited Charlottesville, when I got to their room in the Omni Hotel, both of them sitting at a table by the window, each reading their detective novels. It was a pleasant moment of normality, to see them like that, in the rehab center.

Later, we got to talking about politics, and about how awful the Republicans are. That, too, seemed like a pleasant moment of normality.

I asked my dad today if he and his doctor were talking

about any more chemo. He said he didn't want to do anymore chemo. Apparently the last round of chemo hit him so hard that he preferred to risk the worst just to avoid it.

The doctor seems to be only planning some radiation on my dad's spine. I have not talked to the doctor. I'm not sure what the grand plan is. Perhaps there is no grand plan. I don't like to think about the implications of that very much.

Hope to see you soon.

Hi Paige. I meant to send you this letter a few days ago, but I find it open on my computer screen, which makes me think I never sent it to you?

I am at my folks' house in New Jersey now. I have visited my dad every day this week (he is staying at a rehab clinic, and he undergoes radiation and physical therapy every day). He is still very bright and alert. There is the chance that this visit is my last visit with him, so I'm trying to pack a lot in. We talk mostly about his business, because it seems like the most positive, happy thing we can talk about. He was in the middle of dozens of projects when he lost the ability to walk, and so he has a lot of photos lined up for gallery shows. (He has been a professional photographer for the last 50 years.) He has something like $15,000 worth of prints lying around the house. I want to help him finish these projects. We joke about having "business meetings" at the rehab clinic. I go in and ask him questions and I take notes for an hour. His business is complicated and it is tough for me to learn all the details in just a few days. He tells me where I can find things at the house, and I go home and find them. I'm helping him any way I can.

The rehab clinic is very nice. My parents tell me these things (rehab clinics) are springing up all over the country. Perhaps you've seen them? They are associated with hospitals, but they are cheaper than hospitals, so the insurance companies are pushing them. This particular one, where my dad is at, is set up to feel like a sort of resort hotel, reasonably pleasant. There is a big open room, with a TV, and WiFi, and tables where people can sit, and if you could ignore the people in medical garb, it would feel like a student union at some college campus.

My dad worked through stock photo agencies for most of his life. That meant he got to photograph whatever he felt like and then he'd give the work to the agencies, and they'd sell it for him, in exchange for them keeping either 35% or 50% of the sale (the percent depended on whether the agency had to make all the prints and dupes themselves). The agencies found outlets for his work in advertising, calendars, greeting cards, encyclopedias, etc. My dad made a great living this way, all through the 50s, 60s, 70s, and 80s. In the 90s, the Internet began to change the business, and his sales declined. Over the last 10 years, I've had countless conversations with him about how to revive his business in the era of the Internet. We've had some good brainstorming sessions. At some point he realized that prints, nicely matted and framed, remained a good business, and he began to focus on that. He found outlets in local coffee shops, restaurants, and hospitals. He had some shots of the World Trade Center that became big sellers. I think this year would have been the best year for his business, maybe since 1996, if he hadn't gotten sick.

He is now thinking about fine art galleries. In his youth

and his middle age, I don't think fame was a big concern to him. He would have liked fame, but he did not chase after it. A major photo magazine did a big article on him in 1982, and that could have been a break-out moment for him, but he wasn't committed to chasing after publicity. He was a family man, and he was happy to give a lot of his time to us kids.

Just recently, I think, he has begun to want fame. I think he wants some recognition as one of the great photo crafts-men of his period. This year, in particular, he's thought a lot about trying to get into high-end art galleries in New York. There is a great interest in his early stuff, the photos he did during the 1950s. The commercial work that he did then now seems like classic Americana: restaurants, cars, fashions, all from another era. He's found some galleries in New York that focus on retro nostalgia. If he only had his health, he could pursue this. I find it very sad to think that he simply won't ever get the chance. His early work really deserves a bigger audience.

I was up here in September, and we all went into the city to hit the museums. That may have been my dad's last good month. At that point he had recovered from the radiation and the chemo, and he was feeling good. I suppose that would have been a good time for him to go see the photo galleries himself, but he and his doctors were still thinking he might make a full recovery, so he assumed he could wait until he was feeling even better.

I suppose with illness, every decision is a gamble. Perhaps

that's true of all of one's life, but the reality is much more stark and clear when one is facing a potentially life-ending illness.

I can't even begin to describe how sad I am right now.

Dear Laura,

The other day I was horrified to learn that one of my dad's tumors was up at C3, in his neck. Had it gotten worse, he would have been paralyzed from the neck down. But, from what I can tell, it's gotten better. My dad's arm strength is better. Do you remember last week when he needed our help to move himself up higher in the bed? He's now able to push himself up in the bed. Today I watched him get himself comfortable in the bed, without any help.

It is still extremely sad that he is not walking. But at least his arms seem to be working reasonably well now. That is a positive step.

I've still no idea what his long-term chances are. I worry that, just like last time, as soon as he gets better from this one tumor, he'll start to suffer from another.

Subject: *Working with my dad*
Date: *December 14, 2007*

Note: I had this saved in my "Drafts" folder. I meant to send it to you, but I think I never did?

Dear Misty,

I have been meeting with my dad, at the rehab clinic. Working with him now, this last week, I'm reminded of how little of his work I've seen. Mind you, I've seen a lot of his photos, perhaps 3,000 or 4,000 or 5,000, but he produced 60,000 commercial images during his career, so what I've seen is really a small percentage of the total. In particular, I'm only now seeing much of the work that he did before I was born. The early part of his career.

Apparently this summer, while sick, my dad decided to go through his old work and pick out the very best. He had in mind a gallery show that focused on the 1950s and 1960s. He's been in touch with a gallery in New York City that focuses on nostalgia periods and classic Americana.

Yesterday my dad told me about the pile of images he left behind in his darkroom. His memory for where he's left things is quite good: "Go downstairs into the basement, in my darkroom, turn left after the first table and look at the second, long table. Go to the lightbox in the middle of the table and then look down. You'll see a yellow box, and behind that, there is a pile of negatives. That's the pile I was working on."

I found them exactly where he said they'd be. Today, I took them in to the rehab clinic, so we could go over them together. I need to know what he thinks still has high resale value.

Looking over the work with him was like looking over a history book, with a good historian sitting right next to me, explaining each image.

A car crash in 1951, a Ford and Chrysler smashed to pieces, the owner of the one pointing emphatically to the other.

A snowstorm, and a street full of traffic. This was Flagstaff, Arizona, in 1961, the cars going slowly and the headlights seeming to flicker as the big flakes came down. These were old cars with huge fenders, "space age" cars, the design influenced by the race to the moon.

A redwood forest in the late afternoon; a ray of sunlight coming in at a low angle, piercing the canopy, illuminating a spot in the foreground. This was northern California, in the summer of 1957, the same year that my oldest brother, my parents' first child, was born.

"Do you know what month this photo was taken?" I asked.

"July," he said. "We took a long break after that."

"Why's that?" I asked.

"Lee was born in August."

My mom and dad married in 1953, each pleased they'd found a partner who wanted to travel the world. It took them 4 years to get together the commercial contacts that could pay for their first trip, but once they lined up someone to buy their travel stories and photos, they hit the road. The only thing that would stop them was kids. They promised each other they'd settle down once the first child was old enough to go to kindergarten. That gave them what turned out to be 5 years to be gypsies. Since then, they've done a little traveling almost every year they've been married, but when they speak simply of "the trip," they mean this 5-year trip with which they cemented their life together.

Another photo: an aerial view of midtown Manhattan.

"When is this from?" I asked him.

"1954."

"When did you get your pilot's license?"

"1955."

"What was the name of your partner?"

"Alex von Gliesch."

They were business partners for 3 years, from early 1954 to early 1957. At first, Alex did all the flying. Later, after my dad got his flying license, they would take turns, one of them flying and the other one taking pictures. It was an easy way to make money in those days, when the real estate industry was hot for seeing the land from above.

"You could fly anywhere you wanted to in those days," said my dad. "Now they worry about terrorists, and you'd be shot down if you did half the things that we did then."

The partnership ended when my mom and dad left on their trip. Twenty years later, my dad heard that Alex was in some financial trouble, and then the police came by to ask Dad some questions. Had he seen Alex lately? The police had found Alex's car by a bridge, with a suicide note inside, but the whole river had been dredged and no body had been found, so the suspicion was that Alex had faked his own death. Dad never heard from him, or about him, again.

Another photo: a city draped in Spanish moss. There is Spanish moss on the trees, Spanish moss on the houses, Spanish moss on the power lines. A huge boulevard of cobblestones, surprisingly empty, save for some people walking, and an old streetcar coming up the road, its paint peeling, its wooden sides rotting. This is a sleeping city, New Orleans in 1958. My dad told me they lived a month in the French Quarter, and the grocery where they bought their food was run by a family that still spoke Cajun French as their first language.

Another photo: I see a sleek Mustang in a big city. It's 1964 and the sun is glinting off the sides of multiple skyscrapers, one after the other, off into the distance, a vast canyon of steel; and in the foreground, people going by, a man in a suit holding a briefcase, and next to him two young men with long hair, wearing shirts and pants casually rumpled and dirty. This is Chicago, the same year America got into Vietnam. You can see the people changing then: the different clothes, the different hair, the different lifestyles. America was slowly casting off its gray flannel suit.

Another photo: I see a few tall trees, boughs covered with

snow, and through them, in the distance, a single mountain, filling up the horizon. There are no roads in this picture; no buildings, no cars, no sign of human life. Everything is quiet in the heavy, fresh fallen snow. This is Mount Shasta in 1957.

Another photo: I see several roads converging, all surrounded by tall buildings, some made of brick, others of steel. This is Times Square in 1958. A policeman is directing traffic. On the right, one of the theaters advertises "Elvis Presley in King Creole." There is a fantastic mix of cars and trucks on the streets, some from the 50s, some from the 40s, some possibly from the 30s.

My dad tells me which of these images he thinks will sell, which ones have been printed already, which ones should be scanned into the computer. I take notes. Some of the negatives are nearing the end of their life; they will start to crack and fade soon, some already have. He tells me it's important to find someone who can scan all this work. Over the next ten years, many of these negatives will turn to dust. My dad remembers the kind of film that each shot was taken on, and the archival quality of each brand. His enemy, at this point, was a film produced by Ilford all through the 1950s. It had a terrific tonal range, and at the time he liked it a lot, but starting in the 1990s, these negatives started to peel and crack. These shots, in particular, need to be scanned soon, before the negatives disintegrate. By contrast, most of the films made by Kodak are doing well, and will probably last at least another 20 years.

I'm going to hire someone to start scanning Dad's work. It's a valuable treasure of material, and its commercial value will only increase with time.

Subject: *the present rewrites the past*

Date: *December 20, 2007*

Misty,

There is an old saying that the present rewrites the meaning of the past. Because I've had an intellectual interest in history, I'm used to hearing this saying applied in that context. A revolution breaks out in some country and is interpreted as the beginning of a new and more hopeful era for that country. A few years later, the revolution is crushed and a military dictatorship installed. In retrospect, the revolution is seen as a brief moment of hope, rather than the beginning of a new era.

I haven't often applied this saying to my own life, though now I can see that I soon will. As you know, I was severely ill 12 years ago, in 1995. Crippled with pain, often restricted to my bed, often racing to the emergency room, sometimes uncertain if I was going to live, the doctors doing test after test but still uncertain what was killing me. It was a long time before I was correctly treated, and even longer before I recovered.

For most of that year, I stayed at my parents' house, and my parents, especially my dad, took care of me. I recall my dad staying up with me all night when the pain was so bad that I couldn't sleep. Sometimes he'd read a book to me. He'd bring me something to drink when I was thirsty. When I thought I was facing an immediate crisis, he'd drive me to the local hospital emergency room. Then he'd stay with me, all night, waiting until I was seen by a doctor.

Since that time, I've always thought of 1995 as the worst year of my life. I saw no need to qualify the statement. Few people lose a whole year of their 20s to illness. To say "1995 was the worst year of my life" was to speak the facts as they were, a simple declarative statement to illuminate a simple truth.

My dad is staying at a rehabilitation clinic that is an off-shoot of Jersey Shore Medical hospital, where he received radiation therapy. The clinic has a rule that all visitors must leave by 8 P.M, but these last few nights, they've been nice enough to let me stay all night. I've brought in a voice recorder, and my dad and I stay up late talking about his life, the things he's done, the things he wished he'd done. With his permission, I'm recording it all. He said we should have begun recording our conversations a long time ago. There have been so many good conversations, and so many will be forgotten.

After my dad falls asleep, I read a magazine or I daydream. When he wakes up in the middle of the night, he often has a dry throat, so I get him water, or, if he wants I make him some fresh coffee, using the coffee maker in the staff room that the nurses use. If it seems odd that someone would want to drink coffee at 3 A.M., well, that is my dad. He loves coffee more than anyone else I've ever known.

As the saying goes, the present has a way of rewriting the

meaning of the past. In the future, when I speak of 1995, I will qualify what I say: "1995 was the worst year of my life, except that my dad was there."

My dad is not just my dad, he is also one of my best friends, a fact that I now remind him of often. I sometimes ask him to please live another ten years, and he says he'll do what he can, and then we'll chuckle, but when we are done chuckling we end up crying. He is now, and always has been, my buddy.

Every memory I possess of my dad now seems good to me. Even the worst moments, even the events of 1995, now seem special, because my dad was there. In the future, of course, I will face other crises, and he will not be there to take care of me. I'll miss him.

Subject: *My dad is going downhill*
Date: *December 21, 2007*

Laura,

I'm glad you had a chance to chat with my dad last night, because it might have been the last night anyone could talk to him. He's been delirious all day today. until now, he's only become delirious when he's had a fever, but today he is delirious and for the most part he's had no fever. His fever spiked once in the afternoon, and they gave him Tylenol, but supposedly it did not help.

I get all this information from mom, whom I just talked to on the phone.

When I say delirious, I mean he gets a puzzled face, and then he makes what he thinks is a clever joke, but the words don't quite make sense. Or he tries to ask a question, but again, the words don't make sense.

As an example, this morning when I woke him, I offered him coffee, and he drank it, but his hand shook. He said, "The timing cycles are getting to be double and triple."

I said, "Do you mean the tremors in your arm?"

He said yes. He put the cup down. He said, "I'm surrounded by be-ribboned canoes."

I said, "What?"

He said, "I mean on my blanket. The coffee sloshes."

"Be-ribboned canoes? That's an interesting metaphor."

He squinted up his eyes and thought hard and tried to

put his thoughts together. "I shall get the last drop," he said.

He took a napkin and began cleaning up the coffee he'd spilled on his blanket.

"The multiples of the cycles are getting worse," he said.

"Do you mean the shaking in your hand is getting worse?"

He smiled and said yes, but I don't think he understood the question, and I think he was agreeing just to be agreeable.

It got slowly worse from there.

You were right, I should have brought in the voice recorder every day. I only started recording good conversations with my dad two days ago. I wish I had started weeks ago. I did not think things would go downhill so fast. You were smart to see the risk. My dad was hoping he'd have a positive bounce right after the radiation ended, but that hasn't happened.

At the end of last week my dad seemed stronger than he'd been for some weeks. But that was as strong as he got. Over the weekend he started to slip, and he's been worse every day this week.

I'm just devastated by all of this, and sad, and also angry at myself for not using my voice recorder all year, every time I came up to visit. There is so much time I spent with my dad that I wish I had some recording of.

Subject: *notes from the hospital*
Date: *December 30, 2007*

What follows is a random collection of thoughts about my dad. I began writing it on the night of December 24th. Early on the 25th, my dad had a crisis that caused me to stop writing. I wanted to read this over before I sent it out to you, which is why I'm only sending it out now.

...

As a pre-teen, my father developed a great interest in science. Just a few years later, as a late teen, he subscribed to Scientific American in 1947. My family actually has a complete set of the magazine beginning from that year. Much of my early science education came from my father. I have vivid memories of the many times we would sit down at the kitchen table and he would draw me simple graphs and cartoons to explain the world to me. For instance, when I was 6 years old, I learned some basics about the American Revolutionary War. I was confused why the soldiers stood in thick masses and fired at one another. My father explained how poor the aim was with muskets. He drew an exaggerated cartoon of a barrel and showed me the bullet bouncing awkwardly down the barrel until it left the musket. Then he drew an example of a rifled barrel and how that spun the bullet so the bullet would be stable in flight and go in a straight line. Please note, I've never studied guns, so this explanation, which my father gave me in the 1970s, is the basis of how I understand the history of guns even now.

Eager to ensure that all children had an excellent science education, my father ran for and was elected to the school board, where he served for about 4 years. In this, he also demonstrated to me what it meant to be a good citizen.

I recall one night when I was 7 years old and my dad asked me if I wanted to go stargazing with him. I was very excited by this, partly because it meant that I got to stay up late, but also because I got to do this with him. He'd been a fan of astronomy since his own childhood and he had a lot of books from the 1940s and 1950s (somewhat faded now with yellowing pages) which charted where the stars were in the sky at different times of the night and at different times of the season.

He and I went out into the backyard, which faces the woods. It was pretty dark there, especially back then, before any nearby retail stores had been built. He brought his binoculars and his books and we figured out where certain stars were. I think this was the first time I ever got to use binoculars. New research had determined that Barnard's Star, just 6 light years away, might have a planet just like Earth orbiting around it, so I was keen to figure out just where it was. We talked about the distances to the various stars, and how far a light year was, and we talked about the possibility that humans might be able to travel to the stars one day, far in the future. We talked about how some stars were nearby but dim and how other stars were far away but bright, and how the two stars might end up looking the same, because the more distant star was brighter but its light was dimmed by the distance. My dad told me that 98% of all the stars that I could see were in this galaxy, and that all the other celestial bodies I saw were actually other galaxies, at a great distance.

On the wall of my bedroom, I had a poster of the solar system, and it showed the distance of each planet from the sun. As a kid, I had memorized the exact average distance of each planet's orbit from the sun. He would often read to me the articles in Scientific American, and we would talk about the age of the universe and the why the red shift existed and the theory of the Big Bang. Other articles might have covered things like the structure of an atom, and how there were 104 elements in the universe, and how each element was made up of an atom with a different number of electrons and protons and neutrons.

Because of my dad, I grew up understanding that there were many different scales of distance that were important to science. In some sense, there is a great deal of distance between an electron and the atomic core that it is orbiting, especially if you compare that distance to the closeness of the protons and neutrons at the center. But in another sense, the moon is quite close to the Earth, especially when compared with the size of the galaxy, and both comparisons are true, despite the fact that there is a lot more distance between the moon and the Earth than there is between an electron and its atomic core.

Many parents read to their children at night; my parents did as well. My father had a great respect for my intelligence, so at a young age he let me pick the books. While some children go through a dinosaur craze when they memorize every dinosaur, I went through a World War II phase, when I memorized every war plane from each country in the war. When I was 7 or 8, I signed up for the Military Book Club which was run by Doubleday. The first set of books that I got was the absurdly huge, multi-volume epic Airwar, written by the historian Edward Jablonski. Every night, week after week, month after month, my father read a few pages to me before I fell asleep. I believe it took us more than a year, possibly almost 2 years, to work our way through the entire thing. Occasionally he would stop and share with me some of his own memories of being a teenager during the war. During the war, the U.S. government encouraged teenagers to memorize the silhouettes of German planes, which my father had done with real enthusiasm. He'd once known the supposed strengths and weaknesses of each plane, so for him it was fascinating to go back and learn from a serious military historian which of his memories were correct. And I think it helped me learn how to think logically and strategically, to talk with him about the momentous decisions before each of the leaders and how history might have gone differently if said leaders had made different choices. Considering the pleasure it gave us, my father and I both owe a debt to Edward Jablonski; his book served as the impetus for countless hours of education and discussion.

There are many subjects like that, which I never studied myself, and so my father's explanation remains the bulk of what I know. That's especially true of the electromagnetic spectrum, which my father had memorized. I remember one day we went to the beach and the next day I had a sunburn. I was puzzled why I hadn't felt the heat that burned me and he explained that some forms of radiation don't manifest in what we experience as heat. I was confused, so he sat me down, with paper and pencil, and drew the whole spectrum and explained how different parts of the spectrum affected humans. That's when I learned that there were cosmic rays which pass right through our bodies, and how even that moment, as I sat there listening to him, there was radiation passing through me but not actually touching any of the atoms in my body. That was amazing, but it was also amazing that part of the same spectrum granted us the power of sight and the power of colors. Red light was made of waves 740 nanometers in size, and violet light was 380 nanometers—since he was a photographer, perhaps it is not surprising that he had this part of the spectrum memorized. He also explained that when the sun was close to the horizon, the light passed through more of the atmosphere, which stripped out the high-energy frequencies, and this is why the sky is blue at high noon but can appear yellow or red at sunset.

Many evenings were spent in long discussions about open science questions, such as, why were dogs able to see ultraviolet but humans were not? What evolutionary reason would keep us from having that extra ability?

I've always been quite close to my dad and have regarded him as one of my best friends.

...

When I was a child, and my parents were still in their vigorous prime, they would sometimes talk about how they wished to die. Death was far off and could be seen clearly then, like mountains in the distance. My mom said she'd like to go while asleep: she'd like it if one night, perhaps when she was 104, her heart would simply stop. It made me cry to think that one day Mom would not take care of me, but she assured me that both she and my dad were planning to live very long lives, so I should not worry, because they were going to be around until I myself was quite old. This made me feel a little better, but really I did not want them to ever go. Mom said everyone had to die at some point, and it would be nice to die in one's sleep, as that is the most peaceful way to go. This made sense to me at the time, but since then, I've begun to wonder if such a sudden, unexpected death is really best.

It has the advantage of being easy, but you don't get to say goodbye to people. Saying goodbye is important to me.

My oldest brother, Lee, was 16 in 1973, and that was when he first brought pot home. My dad, 43 at the time, was youthful in spirit, and he tried it out with my brother. My mother refused to ever touch the stuff, since she was opposed to all drugs, but for a few years my brother and my dad both smoked, and Lee's friends regarded our parents as the coolest couple in town. Our house was the preferred spot for teenage parties. Lee became a Republican and an accountant and he denounced his whole rebel past, and when he moved out, the parties stopped and my dad stopped smoking pot. But when my dad spoke of how he'd like to die, he said it would be nice to smoke a lot of pot and take a massive amount of painkillers, and go out peacefully.

I recall driving to Denver once, from the east, and I saw the Rocky Mountains come up like a wall, far out ahead of us, immense and clear in the sunlight. At a distance, one can admire them as a unified whole. However, as I got closer, small hills came up, and then the buildings and the power lines and the smog, and the mountains became harder to see. Death has come up on my dad in the same way. 30 years ago he could envision the ideal death, but this year, when he finally arrived in the neighborhood near death, the view was confused by an endless series of medical tests, chemo, conflicting advice from different doctors, and ever-changing estimates of what his chances of survival were.

In retrospect, it is funny to think of my dad smoking pot. He is so very straight and scientific in all things. But I admire his experimental nature. He is a man who was open to the great variety of experiences that the world had to offer him.

While Dad still had control over his own body, he was never given a moment of clarity about his final end. He may have been waiting for that moment when a doctor said to him, "You are terminal," and then he could have gone home, gathered his family around him, said his goodbyes, smoked some pot, taken a large dose of painkillers, and drifted off to sleep forever. But by the time anyone ever said to him that he had exhausted all treatment options, he was crippled and living in a medical center, and he was taking so many painkillers, and was so worn out from both the pain and the radiation, that he had to rely on my mom to make a lot of the most important decisions. And my mom was not ready to say goodbye to him.

...

I drove to New Jersey on December 1st. Originally, I thought I would visit my dad for 2 weeks, then go home to Virginia, then come back and visit him some more in January. My plans changed only when we realized how fast he was going downhill. When I arrived, he was in the middle of two weeks of radiation therapy. At some point I asked him how much the radiation would do. He said, "It's a long shot, Lawrence. It's a very long shot."

My dad's chances were not good.

"Is it helping?" I asked. "Are you feeling better?"

"Radiation makes you feel worse, at first," he said. "It's a powerful poison. It disrupts the body's biology. You get sick while they give it to you, and you keep getting sick for at least 10 more days after it is over. Then, maybe, you might get a little bounce."

The cancer has moved with astonishing speed. Even the doctors have been surprised. In November of 2006, Dad began to wonder if his ability to swallow had grown worse. He has had a slight problem swallowing since childhood. I recall, when I was very young, there was a time that the whole family was at a restaurant and Dad got up and went to the bathroom for over an hour. My mom sent my older brother to check on him. A bit of food had got stuck on the way down, and my dad was uncomfortable. After another hour, the problem simply went away. This happened somewhat often, and people used to ask my dad if he was choking. The question annoyed him, mostly because he had to repeat himself so often: The problem was lower than that, there was never any risk to his air passageways. His problem swallowing was closer to his stomach. In 2003, for some reason, Dad had a flare-up, and things were worse for a while. But then it resolved itself and he was fine.

In January of 2007, my dad began to suspect that he was facing a new problem, rather than a worsening of the old problem. Since Mom and Dad had planned to spend February traveling around in Florida, Dad made an appointment with a doctor and scheduled it for March. In March, he underwent some tests and was told he had cancer of the esophagus. In May, he began treatment. By July, the lump his throat was gone, but he was told the cancer had spread to his lymph nodes. In August, he tried another round of chemo.

The multiple treatments he underwent during the summer left him exhausted and weak, so his doctor told him he should take some time off from treatment, regain his weight and strength. For September, Dad tried to simply relax, eat well, and get some exercise.

In October, Dad tried another round of chemo. Because the disease had spread, the doctor was trying the strongest stuff possible, and it made my dad very sick. The basic idea with chemo is that you take poison and you hope it kills the cancer cells before it kills you. Since cancer cells are fast-growing, they are usually more vulnerable to poison than normal cells. But not always.

Dad began to feel a weakness in his legs, which he and the doctor initially thought was the fault of the chemo. The doctor told him to take another month off.

During the first half of November, Dad's legs rapidly got weaker. On the 19th, he fell down and could not get up. Mom called 911 and Dad was taken to the emergency room.

X-rays revealed that he now had two tumors on his spine. One of the tumors was low down in his thoracic area, and it was interfering with his ability to walk. The other tumor was up at the C3 vertebrate, in his neck, and it was beginning to effect the strength and dexterity of his arms.

The medical center he is at focuses on physical rehabilitation. The center is mostly for those who've just been through successful surgery and who therefore need some therapy to get back to normal (people who have complications during their surgeries don't come here; they go to the Intensive Care Unit in the hospital where they were operated on). A typical resident of this facility is a senior citizen who has just had hip replacement surgery, and who is now building up the muscles around their new fake hip bone.

Dad didn't feel the radiation was doing him any good, but, from my perspective, it clearly did. When I first arrived in New Jersey, he was having some trouble using his arms, but by the end of the radiation, the strength and dexterity of his arms had seemingly returned to normal. In the physical therapy sessions, with two parallel bars to help hold him up, he regained the ability to take a few tentative steps. It struck me that, with enough time, he would be able to walk again.

...

The Earth is 4.5 billion years old and life on Earth is at least 3.5 billion years old, but for most of the Earth's history, life existed only in the form of single-celled organisms. The Cambrian Revolution began 560 million years ago, and this was when the first multi-celled creatures evolved. Cancer has been a problem ever since. In the most general terms, cancer can be thought of as the desire of a cell in a multi-celled organism to revert to the primordial autonomy that was the norm for the first 3 billion years of life on Earth.

During the Cambrian Revolution, some organisms evolved from one cell into organisms that had 10 cells, then 100 cells, then 1,000, then a million, and then a billion, and then a trillion. I've read that the average adult human body has roughly 30 to 50 trillion cells. As organisms became more complex, mechanisms evolved that helped individual cells behave as helpful pieces of a larger whole. For instance, in humans, each cell has the p53 gene which regulates cell division. A cell cannot reproduce until the p53 gene has created a protein (the tumor suppressing protein) which, essentially, checks to see that the cell is reproducing in a healthy way. Sadly, the p53 gene can be damaged by viruses or toxic chemicals or a number of other environmental assaults. But the p53 gene is not the only mechanism in the cells that stops cancer; rather, each cell has multiple checks on its own growth. It is only when all of these mechanisms have been damaged or destroyed that cells become cancerous.

I have often wondered how my dad got sick. It is rare for

non-smokers to get cancer of the esophagus, and except for the pot that he tried for a few years in the 70s, my dad never smoked. Certainly, he never smoked cigarettes. He did spend a good portion of his life developing photos in his darkroom, and I suppose it is possible that one or more of the chemicals he dealt with might have had carcinogenic properties. It's not very likely though, or darkroom photography, as a profession, would be associated with high levels of cancer.

We will never know for sure.

...

We are getting to know the nurses here.

Nurse Kathy, for instance, is in her early 30s, physically fit and exuding confidence. Her competence can be assumed from her manner, and by the rapport she establishes with each patient. Her professionalism seems impervious to blemish, no matter the multiple competing demands that a patient, and the members of the patient's family, put on her.

For instance, one night when Dad wasn't feeling well, we asked her to come in and talk to him. We were trying to be careful, so we asked her to check one thing after another: his temperature, his blood-oxygen level, his pulse, etc. Sometimes Mom and I were at odds, with me asking for more tests and Mom trying to get the nurse to go away. Mom wants everyone to like her, so she dislikes pushing the staff too hard, but I feel like we've an obligation to defend Dad's health, even if that means we are seen as overly demanding. Afterwards, when nurse Kathy was leaving, I apologized that we asked so much of her.

"I am so sorry about all the requests," I said. "We just get very worried about Dad."

"Please don't apologize," said nurse Kathy. "This is my job. This is what I'm here for."

"You're doing an amazing job," said my mom. "And we're proud of you." My mom, an early feminist, was good about saying supportive things to women, especially in professional positions.

"Thank you," said nurse Kathy. "But, really, I'm here to help you. This is what I'm supposed to do."

"It must be tough for you," I said, "to have to negotiate all the different personalities in a family."

"Please don't worry about me," she said. "Focus on yourselves. I mean it. What you're going through is tough. Don't worry about me."

Quite different is nurse Sandy, the only one of the nurses who will openly show her exasperation with us. She is in her late 20s, which perhaps makes her the youngest of the nurses that we speak with here. She is pretty in the most conventional American sense, with blond hair, blue eyes, and a fairly thin figure. She looks like she grew up on a farm out in Iowa, and she also tends to use words like "shucks" and "darn." She is the morning nurse; her shift starts at 7 AM. I recall at one point, when she was doing her morning rounds, pushing her cart slowly down the hall and taking meds into each room, to each patient, I went out and told her that my dad was in some discomfort. She said, "Okay," and gave no other reaction. I didn't know what to make of that, but I went back into my dad's room.

15 minutes passed and she did not come in. I went back into the hall and found her and repeated that my dad was in some discomfort. She didn't look at me, but shrugged her shoulders and, with obvious exasperation, said, "I've got a lot of patients to take care of!" In contrast to Kathy's confidence, Sandy always gives the impression that she is overwhelmed by her responsibilities.

Basically, nurse Kathy is the nurse you always hope to have when you're in the hospital, and nurse Sandy is the nurse you pray won't be assigned to you.

...

Each day, my mom would insist that my dad get in his wheelchair and come out to the main room—a pleasant room with a lot of tables, a bookcase, a magazine rack, and a big TV. The room feels like the student union of a university, except the people in it are older. In this room, my dad and I would sit at a table and get our work done.

We were working our way through a big pile of negatives, and he was telling me when and where each image was taken, and whether he thought it had high value. There was an image of the Garden State Parkway from 1959, and another of Chicago in 1964, and another of the redwoods in northern California from 1957. I held up another one, which looked like New York City, earlier than the others, and asked when it was from.

"It's from 1980," he said.

I was puzzled. I looked at the image. There were a bunch of cars from either the late 1940s or early 1950s on a New York street.

"Dad, look at the image again," I said. "When is it from?"

"1980," he said.

"Dad, what are you talking about? Check out the number that you assigned this image. It's from one of your early series."

He seemed puzzled by this fact, and also by the fact that he couldn't make sense of the date, or even why 1980 was the wrong date.

I'd never before seen my dad miss a date like that. For my dad, as with me, a date is a primary category. Chronology is important to both of us, an essential tool through which we organize our mental maps of the world. I thought Dad was having a "senior moment," but I didn't say this aloud, as it would be rude. Also, it was possible that the painkillers were playing tricks on his mind, making it harder for him to think clearly. I was surprised by the incident, as I'd never seen him slip like that before, but I was willing to move on to the next image.

I did not know it then, but that slip was the beginning of a dementia that would spring up the next week and sweep away his chances of making clear decisions regarding his own fate.

...

The next day I brought in more photos to go over, but Dad found it difficult to concentrate and we had to give up after about 30 minutes. He also said his body felt uncomfortable. At the time I thought it was because he'd been doing extra sessions of physical therapy, which was wearing him down but concurrently making him stronger. The reality, which I did not know then, is that he was beginning to feel the onset of a new wave of cancer.

...

When I saw Dad on Sunday the 16th, he didn't feel like working. Instead, he and my mom and I all had dinner together. When I arrived, they were both out in the main room at one of the small, private tables and we all ordered dinner. The food was surprisingly good. When I thought about us all sitting there, having dinner at a table together, the moment felt wonderfully normal.

...

The next day, Monday the 17th, when I arrived at the rehab center in the afternoon, my dad was completely disoriented and largely unable to speak. When he did speak, his words were complete nonsense. My mom was sitting with him at one of the tables in the main room. Most days, they would sit together and read the newspaper or novels. On this day, however, he was unable to read, and was, in fact, seemingly unaware of his surroundings. My mom was sitting in her chair and praying for him.

"What's wrong with Dad?" I asked.

"I don't know," said mom. She had her eyes closed and had reached across the corner of the table so she could hold his hand.

"Is there a doctor around?" I asked.

"No," she said.

"A nurse?"

"They won't know anything. We need to ask a doctor."

"When will the doctor be in?"

"On Wednesday."

"Dad can't stay like this for two days. We need to get someone to check him."

"They can't check him until Wednesday. Wait until Wednesday. The doctor will be here."

"Should we take Dad to the hospital?"

"No! Do you know what that would mean? They would have to transfer him in this freezing cold, in an ambulance, and he'd have to sit in the emergency room for hours, and then he'd been seen by a doctor who knows nothing about his case."

I saw Kathy standing by her cart, filling out some paperwork, so I went over to her.

"Excuse me, nurse Kathy? My dad doesn't seem to be doing well. Can you come over and look at him?"

"Of course. Give me one second."

I went back to the table and Kathy came over a moment later.

"How are you doing, Ralph?" she asked.

My dad was staring at the table. He grimaced. He squinted. He made no sound. He did not look up at her.

She took his pulse, which was fine. Then she pulled out a little device called a Pulsox, which could measure the oxygen level in his blood. The device had two parts: a small clip that went over one of his fingers, and a hand-held part that had a LED screen that read out numbers. It seems like a magic trick that a small clip on one's finger can read one's blood-oxygen level. As long as the number was between 90 and 100, my dad was okay. My dad's number was 94.

"His pulse and his oxygen level are okay," said Kathy.

"What would cause him to become so disoriented?" I asked.

She thought for a moment.

"He could have a fever," she said. "I'll take his temperature."

She got another device off her cart. This was a handheld device, one end of which could be put in the ear. It almost instantly read out Dad's temperature: 102 F.

"He does have a fever," she said. "I'll give him some Tylenol."

The effects of the Tylenol were dramatic. Over the next hour, Dad came back to his senses, pretty much completely, save for some drowsiness that I attributed to painkillers. There was a magic moment when he looked at us and realized we were there.

A while passed and then I asked him how he was feeling.

"It's amazing," he said. "I'd been thinking that I was at a facility run by the CIA. They had a sinister plan to use me. We were in Connecticut. I had a sense of dread and panic. The place was evil. Then suddenly I was here, and I saw you two. I was very surprised that I was here, and that you were here."

"Incredible."

"Really. I've never had such an experience, nor would I have thought I could recover from it with something as weak as Tylenol."

At the time, I found it surprising that Dad would have such intense hallucinations when his fever was only 102. I thought that maybe fevers had more impact on old people, so that a fever of 102 was hitting him like a fever of 106 would hit me. Or perhaps the painkillers were making it easier for him to hallucinate.

Kathy checked back with us after an hour and was glad to see that Dad was doing better.

"But what could be causing the fever?" I asked.

Kathy thought about it a moment.

"Sometimes UTIs cause fever and change of mental status in older people," she said. "Ralph, we should take a urine sample, just to be sure."

We all agreed it was good to check, so Kathy provided a container for urine and Dad wheeled himself to the bathroom and produced a sample that could be sent out and checked for urinary tract infections. Kathy took it and said the results would be back tomorrow.

"Will the doctor prescribe antibiotics?" I asked.

"Yes," she said. "If the results come back positive, he'll probably prescribe antibiotics."

I was thinking that whatever the problem was, it should be chased aggressively, since these kinds of infections can get out of control among older people, and Dad had enough problems to deal with.

We were all terribly innocent at that point. We didn't know the horror that was soon to come.

...

When I first came up to New Jersey, Laura suggested that I take my digital voice recorder in when I go to see Dad. As soon as she suggested this, I became hooked on the idea. Before Dad died, I wanted to spend a few weeks with him going over his life, and our life. I wanted to talk about the good times, and the bad times, and I wanted us to recall, together, how close we'd been. I also wanted to capture some of his travel stories, which I love. I also wanted to capture some of his alternative interpretations of scientific theories like the Big Bang and the red shift. (He worried that scientists were engaging in religious theory by referring to the Big Bang but not trying to describe what existed prior to it.) Some of these were conversations we'd had many times before, but I wanted to capture them forever on my recorder, so that I wouldn't have to depend on my own weak, fast-fading memory. I imagined that over the weeks I might capture hundreds of hours of my dad talking and when he was gone, whenever I wanted to remember what he'd meant to me, I could listen to the recordings and recall him fondly.

However, I was disorganized and somehow delayed bringing in my voice recorder for most of the first 3 weeks that I was in New Jersey. As things turned out, the first night that I brought it was to be the last night that my dad was wholly lucid, and I only captured about 2 hours of us having the kinds of nostalgic conversations that I thought we might spend weeks having.

Of all the mistakes I have ever made, there are very few that I will regret as much as this one.

...

On Tuesday, the test results came back. My dad did not have a UTI. The nurse said they would draw blood and send that out for more tests. There was discussion of moving him to a hospital, so that the tests could be done more quickly. But there was a sense that Dad was comfortable at the current spot, and we knew the staff, so he stayed at the rehab clinic, despite the fact that I found it frustrating how slowly everything moved.

My dad had a cold, and someone suggested maybe it was pneumonia. Since this is a serious killer among older people, the idea made me frantic. Yet somehow, the staff didn't draw blood until 5 AM on Wednesday morning, and no results came back that day. He continued to have an occasional fever that would spike and leave him delirious. I kept asking nurses to check his temperature and to give him Tylenol when he had a fever.

Since my dad started having episodes, he could no longer take care of himself when he woke up in the middle of the night. He could no longer be depended upon to get himself water, or signal a nurse when he needed help. So I started staying overnight. Each day I've been coming in at 5 P.M. and staying until 9 AM. He says it is very comforting to wake up in the middle of the night and see me sitting next to his bed.

...

On the evening of Thursday the 20th, we had not yet heard about any results of the tests, and Dad was still not being treated for whatever was causing his fever. I asked a nurse to come in. Nurse Carol was on duty that night, the oldest and perhaps most experienced of the nurses.

"We're looking for some information," I said. "We're trying to figure out what's going on. My dad's had a fever all week. We thought we'd hear back about some test results by now."

"Um, listen," she said. "You look frantic. Is there a partic-ular reason why you might appear that way?"

She came over and said this very directly to me. I could

tell that I was losing credibility with her because I seemed agitated about the lack of information. From this, I learned something important: No matter what happens, I must never look frantic again. The staff can ignore me if I look frantic.

"I'm so sorry," I said. I smiled and tried to look relaxed and non-frantic. "I'm just worried about my dad, is all. He's had a fever and I was hoping the cause of it would be treated."

Something I said gave her a bit of a clue about where I was coming from. Then an expression came over her face, which, if I read it correctly, was something like, "The poor sap! No one has told him the truth yet!" Her manner changed completely. She started talking in a soft voice, like she might talk to a child.

"Well," she said. "Your dad is going to decline. I'm sorry to say, this is part of the natural process of how this disease progresses. It's very sad, but this is expected."

We talked a little bit about how the process worked out. I asked her how long my dad had, and she said no one could possibly know. When I thought that he didn't have much longer, I started to cry. I explained to her that I hadn't been able to get much information from my folks, so I was curious what was going on. She said that my dad's doctor, Dr. Patel, was present in the building tonight, and she could send him in, if we wished. I said that would be ideal. She went out to get him.

Dr. Patel came in, along with the head nurse, a woman named Ms. Kong. Dr. Patel spoke with my father for a moment, and then he addressed all of us. His manner was gentle and informative. I was trying to find out if there were any other treatment options. He largely confirmed that all treatment options were exhausted. "A person can only go through so many cycles." He did make the mistake of saying that the next day he would talk to Dr. Briggs, who'd overseen the radiation, to see if there were any other treatments. I believe Dr. Patel said this simply because the truth was so brutal, and yet this was a case where being brutal would have been helpful.

The staff, over and over again, kept trying to be gentle with us and so they kept phrasing things as if there was still something that might be done for Dad. They were underestimating how strong our denial was and how badly we wanted to have some reason for hope. What we needed was a moment when someone simply said, "It's over. Say your goodbyes." But the staff was never quite that explicit, because they thought being that explicit would be rude.

All the same, Dr. Patel did mostly leave us with the impression that it was over. Dad was ahead of us, in that he had already understood this. My mom and I were crying, and even the head nurse began to cry. For some reason, I was honored by the fact that she would be moved to tears. She must see a fair number of people die.

They turned to leave, and they said they'd send in the social worker to talk to us about the actual details of the dying. For my mom and dad and I, it was time to say goodbye.

My mom, crying uncontrollably, said, "I hope you had a

nice life."

"I did, honeybear," he said.

"Dad," I said. "I want you to stick around for another ten years."

"I'd like that, too, Lawrence," he said.

"You're my best friend," I said.

"Thank you, Lawrence."

"You're my best buddy," I said.

"You're my best buddy, too," he said.

He really is. And I want to be a good buddy to him, while he is dying. Part of that means protecting him from pain, and a lot of what I've done over the last few days, and will continue to do, is based on my desire to be a good buddy.

We talked about his work and its importance. I wanted to reassure him that he would not be forgotten.

"We're going to keep promoting your work, Dad."

"Thank you, Lawrence."

I wanted to cheer him up, so I said, "Twenty years from now, you are going to be famous." That could turn out to be true, of course.

"That is pleasant to think about," he said. "I wanted people to know that there is a lot of value there, in the old prints, so I'm glad you and I had the chance to talk about."

"It's a treasure trove," I said. "And we will keep promoting it."

Then he was worried about me: "But you go live your own life, too. You could spend your whole life just looking at those old photos, but then one day you'd find the calendar is running out on you."

"I'll live my own life, Dad." I wanted to reassure him that I was going to have a good life. "I'm going to have a great life."

But I know that most of his life he wondered why he wasn't breaking out into the big leagues, and these last 4 or 5 years, and especially this last year that he's been sick, he's been thinking that he never achieved the level of attention that he deserved.

At some point, the social worker came in to talk to us about death. She asked Dad if he wanted to sign a Do Not Resuscitate and a Do Not Hospitalize order. We all knew what a DNR was, and Dad said yes. He said yes to the DNH without really thinking about it. I'd never heard of a Do Not Hospitalize order before, but the social worker mentioned it in the same breath as the DNR, so we went along with it thinking that it was sort of the same thing. We made a bad mistake by not asking more questions.

Later on, I began to think that we should have taken Dad to a hospital, where they might be better set up to manage the pain of someone who was dying. But the social worker assured us that the rehab facility would be able to manage his pain and keep him comfortable as he died. I later realized that "keep him comfortable" means one thing to a medical professional and something quite different to someone with little experience with hospitals. For us, the phrase "keep him comfortable" meant simply "keep him free of pain." Others might laugh at my ignorance, but up until now I've always thought that, given enough painkillers, a person could die without pain. Apparently, this isn't true.

Dad's main concern was that he be able to end his life without pain. He said that if things got really bad, he'd like to be able "to hit an escape button and get out of here." That is an exact quote which I take from one of my recordings. The social worker kept saying over and over again, "We can keep him comfortable." This turned out to be a lie. They have not been able to manage his pain. This is partly because the nurses are afraid to call the doctor—they risk losing credibility every time they do; they risk appearing "frantic" in the eyes of the doctor. But they can't increase my dad's pain medication without getting the doctor's permission. Thus, every day, my dad's pain gets ahead of the medication, and every day, I have to pressure the nurses to call the doctor.

What exactly did my dad mean when he said he wanted "an escape button"? At the time, I was assuming he wanted an easy way to die. I guess we all should have thought more clearly about that. Suicide is illegal in New Jersey, but we could have managed it, so long as we got him out of this place and took him home, and so long as he was still lucid enough to take the painkillers on his own. But he knew that speaking of this option in blunt terms would hurt my mom's feelings, so he was not explicit about what he meant. The other possibility for an "escape option" would be a moment that he could tell the staff, "I want to be unconscious from here on out." I wish we'd gotten a commitment from the staff for this option. Instead we got a bunch of euphemisms about "keeping him comfortable," none of which were fully honest.

Later, Mom went home and it was just me and Dad. I asked again if it was okay if I recorded all our conversations, and he said we should have started recording our conversations a long time before. From here on, I had my voice recorder on for nearly every encounter with my dad, my mom, or any nurse. I'd originally hoped to capture weeks of conversations with my dad about his life, but what I ended up with was day after day of dialogue arising from the crisis around his dying.

You cannot imagine how sad this makes me.

...

On Friday the 21st, they moved Dad to a private room. This was in recognition of the fact that he needed someone to look after him during the night. A private room made it easier for them to authorize me to stay overnight. It was a big room, originally designed for two beds, but now with just one bed. Where the other bed would have been was, instead, a big, plush fold-out chair. A visiting overnight guest would certainly have an easier time sleeping in that chair than in the simple utilitarian chairs I'd be dozing off in for the whole week. Here, in this room, my dad had sole control of the TV, and my mom and I had more room to spread out our stuff.

Also on the 21st, my dad said he was short of breath. When the nurses checked his oxygen level, they found it had dipped below 90 for the first time, to 88. They brought in a machine and set it up in the room. This is a clever machine, it has a small bottle of distilled water attached to it, which it runs through electrolysis to produce some oxygen. This isn't a high-pressure source of oxygen, like being hooked to an oxygen tank would be. Instead, it supplies a small dose of pure oxygen, and it is perfect for giving someone a small oxygen boost, like what my dad needed now. Also, since the oxygen is created and then immediately inhaled; there is no pure oxygen left floating around. Therefore it is much safer than, say, having a big tank of oxygen just sitting there in the room. The machine attached to my dad through a small plastic tube that could be looped around his two ears and left just under the nose, pointing up into it, blowing oxygen. All in all, this was fairly comfortable and non-invasive. The tube didn't really go up his nose vertically; it just sat there under his nose and blew a little oxygen.

I was shocked by how much my dad had gone downhill in just one day, and I was shocked that he was now delirious more often than he was lucid. For the first time, he had a period of delirium though he had no fever—that is to say, he was now having delirium that was arising purely as a result of the cancer.

Dad had spoken of wanting "an escape button," but it now struck me that things were getting bad fast and we might need to plan how exactly that escape button was going to happen. At one point, I took my mom aside and asked what the strategy was. Was she thinking of finding some alternative therapies, or was it time, perhaps, to take Dad home? She misunderstood me. She said it would be too expensive to take Dad home. I was thinking that we would only take him home if he wanted to end everything, but it seemed too brutal to say this out loud. She also talked a bit about herbal remedies and immune boosters. I'm not sure if she was serious about this, or if she was saying such things for form's sake. She said that Western, allopathic medicine destroyed people's immune systems and that Dad's only hope was if we could build his immune system up. I asked her if she had a plan for that, but she said she wasn't sure how to sneak such a remedy into a place like this. Again, I'm not sure she was really serious. Her own emotions were adjusting to the reality of his dying, and it could be that she was politely asking for time to adjust.

I left the subject alone because I figured we could take it up a few days later. This was my second big mistake.

...

By Sunday the 23rd, my dad was delirious most of the time. I think the saddest moment was when he woke up in the middle of the night and forgot that there was anything wrong with his legs. I'd been sitting next to his bed, thinking about our life and what we'd shared, and suddenly his eyes popped open.

"Lawrence!"

"Dad?"

He looked around then back at me. He seemed frustrated and scared.

"Let's go," he said.

"Where do you want to go?"

"Let's go!"

"Where do you want to go, Dad?"

"We've got to get out of here!"

For the last 2 or 3 days, he'd developed a panic about being in that bed. Especially when he was delirious, he began to associate the bed with death. He seemed to think that if he could get out of the bed, and escape the rehab clinic, he'd be able to live; but if he stayed there, then death would find him. I had a hard time thinking of what to say to him. I wanted to allay his panic, yet he really couldn't go anywhere.

"Dad, we should probably stay here."

He shook his head. He threw back all the blankets and moved toward the edge of the bed. He was startled by his own body.

"Lawrence, why are my legs not working?"

"Dad, the cancer caused some damage to your spinal column, which has damaged your ability to walk. You just went through two weeks of radiation therapy to heal your spine. You need to stay here at least until your spine begins to heal."

He shook his head no. He was determined to go. With his hands, he grabbed his legs and tried to move them to the edge of the bed. I jumped up.

I jumped up. "Dad, please be careful. I don't want you to hurt yourself."

"We've got to go!"

He was in a panic.

"Dad, I could get an aide to help you into a wheelchair, but, the last time you were in a wheelchair, your oxygen level crashed."

His legs were too heavy for him to move, so he gave up, frustrated. He fell back in the bed.

"Lawrence?" His voice is very tired and quiet now.

"Yes, Dad?"

"I hurt."

"Where do you hurt?"

"My back."

"Should we roll you a bit, Dad?"

"Okay."

I suspect a new tumor is growing on my dad's tailbone. It has been causing him agonizing pain. We've learned that sometimes just rolling side to side can relieve the pressure a bit. I took his arm and put my arm around his body and I helped him roll onto his left side.

"Does that help, Dad?"

"Good."

We held that position for a moment.

"Okay," he said.

We rolled back to the middle, then we rolled to the other side. We did this several times. It seemed to help with his pain. After that, he was worn out. He sat there a while, mostly reclining, and then he started to doze. I sat next to him. I wanted to go out to the main hall where they have a machine that makes Green Mountain coffee, good stuff, but every time I moved, his eyes opened again. He was on the edge of sleep, but he was not sinking into it.

A while later, his eyes opened and he looked right at me.

"Lawrence?" His voice was very weak.

"Yes, Dad?"

"I... I hurt."

"Where does it hurt, Dad?"

He shook his head. He was miserable.

"All over."

"I'll get the nurse."

I went to the nurses station. No one was there. I looked down each hallway. No one could be seen. In the main dining room, there was an aide who was sleeping at one of the tables. I waited for a while, but I didn't want to leave Dad alone for long, so after a few minutes I went back. He was looking at me hopefully when I came in.

"I'm still looking for the nurse, Dad."

"I... I hurt."

"I know, Dad. I'm sorry. I will find a nurse."

I went back out. This facility is not set up for people like Dad who have emergencies. This facility is mostly for people recovering from successful surgeries, people who can, for the most part, take care of themselves. In a typical hospital, especially in an ICU unit, there will be one nurse for every 3 patients. In a crisis, for a short period, one nurse might have to watch 5 or 6 patients. But here, there is one nurse for every 16 patients. (The low staff-to-patient ratio is one thing that makes these facilities relatively inexpensive, which is one reason the hospitals and insurance companies have been pushing them.) Sometimes it's quite hard to find a nurse.

I waited at the nurses station until a nurse came back. This was nurse Maricel, a woman from the Philippines, who was very competent.

"Excuse me. Could you come see my father in room 101? He is in pain."

"Hmm." She checked the clock. "Let me see when he last got pain medicine."

Maricel grabbed a gigantic 3-ring binder packed full of documentation and pulled it out. I assumed my dad's chart was somewhere inside there. Later I noticed that his name was on the side of this binder, so the whole thing was devoted just to him. I had to assume this held his whole medical history, back to the first tests for cancer in March.

"Yes," she said. "It's been 4 hours. I can bring him something."

I went back to my dad's room.

"I hurt!" he said. His voice was weak but he was in great pain now.

"The nurse is coming, Dad."

He was dozing in and out, but when he was awake, he was groggy.

"Help!" he said.

"Hang in there, Dad."

His eyes pleaded with me. He seemed to feel that I wasn't understanding how much pain he was in.

"Help!"

"The nurse is coming, Dad."

"Hurry!"

The nurse came in and gave him a dose of Roxanol. It was fast-acting. After 5 minutes, he felt some relief. After 20 minutes, he almost dozed off. Then he woke again, startled. I believe he was trying to keep himself awake, because he feared that if he fell asleep he would die.

"Lawrence?" His voice was very weak.

"Yes, Dad?"

"Let's..."

"Dad?"

"Let's get out of here? Okay?"

"Where do you want to go?"

"Out."

"Dad, I'm not sure I understand where we are going to go."

"I'm worried... I'm worried that I'm wasting...my last chance. This could be my last chance."

I found it very difficult to think of what to say to that. It seemed overly brutal to say, simply, "Dad, you must stay here and die. There is nothing that can be done to help you. We have chosen to await death here." I couldn't possibly say it, but I hate being dishonest with my dad. I've noticed that sometimes the aides will come in, and when he cries out in pain they will give him false assurances, like, "You'll be better soon." (The nurses almost never do this, just the aides.) When he is lucid, or even semi-lucid, this kind of thing frustrates him profoundly, so I never indulge it. But I find that if I avoid lying and if I avoid the brutal truth, I'm left with very little I can say.

"Dad, if we leave here, your oxygen level will crash. We need to be sure that you're getting enough oxygen."

"Lawrence... When I feel... This could be my last chance. I need to get out of here. When I feel like this... We can go... We need to be careful... I'm worried... I'm worried..."

"I know, Dad. I'm very sorry. I'd do anything I could to help you. Anything. But I don't know what to do."

"What if...this is my last chance? We need...to do something."

"I'm so sorry, Dad. I love you with all my heart. I'd do anything I could for you."

"I want to live."

For me, this was simply the most heartbreaking thing he could have said. I wanted him to live, too. I could not fully believe that he was dying. It seemed unfair to me that there should be nothing we could do.

"Aw! Dad! I want you to live, too!"

I started crying again. I took his hand.

"I want you to live another 20 years, Dad. If there were anything I could do to make it happen, I'd do it. I just don't know what to do."

"I want...to live."

"Dad. I'm so sorry. I'm so sorry. I love you so much. You're my best buddy. I wish there were something I could do."

He thought to himself for a while. His eyes started to close. He dozed off again.

Suddenly he was awake again. I felt his hand tighten on mine and I looked at him.

"The yellow..." he said.

"What, Dad?"

"The yellow."

He was completely delirious now.

"What's yellow?"

"Get rid of all the yellow."

"Okay."

"The boards?"

"Yes?"

"All of it?"

"Okay."

"The eggs?"

"Okay."

"You will?"

"Yes, Dad, sure."

"Get rid of all the yellow."

"Okay."

"And then the white."

"Okay."

"Get rid of all the white."

"Okay."

"I mean, with the eggs."

"Okay."

"You're sure?"

"Yes, Dad."

"Good."

He stared at me for a while, waiting for me to act. At one point, he shook my hand, as if to say, "Get a move on it! What are you waiting for? This is urgent!" I smiled and nodded my head.

"I promise," I said.

He nodded, happy that I was going to do it. He looked around the room. Sometimes he blinked in surprise at something in the air. I believe he was seeing hallucinations, because last week, when he was still mostly lucid, he told me in the middle of one of our conversations that he had just hallucinated a blanket flying through the air.

He dozed off again, and I thought he was going to get some sleep. I stayed by him, still holding his hand. After a while he woke up again. He was in some pain.

"Lawrence?"

"Yes, Dad?"

"Why am I covered in sand?"

He seemed to be looking at the white blankets that were covering him.

"This isn't sand, Dad. These are blankets. They are to keep you warm. Are you too warm?"

"Yes."

I wasn't sure if this was true. I've learned that when he gets delirious, he tends to say yes to every question I ask him.

"Dad, are you too cold?"

"Yes."

I was hoping that physical action might allow him to communicate with me about what he actually needed. I removed one of the blankets.

"Is this better, Dad?"

"Yes."

That didn't tell me anything. I started to put the blanket on him again.

"No!" he said. He waved it away. That told me something. I folded it up and stored it in the closet.

I sat with him through the night. He often woke up and made a face that I've learned indicates dryness of the throat.

Sometimes he couldn't speak, he could only look pained, and he scrunched up his mouth. I brought a cup of water to his lips and he took a sip, then rinsed his mouth with the water, then swallowed. Then he went back to dozing.

Somewhere around 3 or 4 AM, he slipped into a deep sleep. I figured he was going to be okay for the night and I allowed myself to shut my eyes for a while.

I woke up a while later. Dad was gasping for air and looking panicked. To my horror, I realized that he had removed the breathing tube from his nose. I jumped up and put it back in.

"Dad! You've got to keep this on! You understand? You've got to keep this on."

He nodded his head, but I wasn't certain he understood me.

"Get me out," he said. His voice was weak; he spoke in a whisper.

"Are you having shortness of breath?"

"Get me out!"

He was very agitated. At times when he wakes up delirious, he has something like a panic attack—his heart races very fast, which then makes it harder for him to breathe.

"I'll get the nurse."

"Get me out of here!"

I went out to the nurses station. "My dad is having trouble sleeping."

The nurse checked my dad's chart.

"Well," said the nurse, "He's not due for pain medication for 2 more hours, but we can give him Xanax to calm him and help him sleep."

"Okay."

I went back to my dad's room. He had dozed off again. The nurse came in, we woke Dad, and we gave him the Xanax. Then the nurse left.

"Get me out," he started again.

"Dad, we should stay here. Your oxygen level will crash if we go anywhere. Let's wait for a little bit, and then you can catch your breath."

"Get me out."

It took a while for the Xanax to have any effect. Then he slept again, more deeply than before.

...

It's 5 A.M. right now on December 24th. I have been pacing back and forth in the room, in the hallway just outside the door, away from where my dad is. I think best when I pace. I'm trying to foresee the consequences of his death; I'm trying to finally get ahead of the curve. It has been a year full of ambushes; I'm hoping to get to the point where we can see the next disaster coming and avoid it. For instance, the funeral. How much will it cost? And the costs of living: What will Mom do? Is the mortgage paid off? How much is Dad's health insurance covering, and how much debt are we running up? I'll have to talk to Lance about that. We both have good-paying jobs, so perhaps we can split the cost.

I'm too tired to stay on my feet, so I'm sitting down in the chair next to my dad's bed. I can feel myself beginning to doze off... I hope that I'm close enough to his bed that if he stirs I'll wake up.

My thoughts no longer occur in any order. I wonder if there are treatment options out there, unknown to us. I wonder how much time it would take us to track them down. I wonder how much time Dad has left. I guess the radiation didn't work though I wish... Wait a minute, didn't Dad say he would get worse after the radiation? He said that the first time, back in July, he actually continued to get more sick for 10 days after the radiation. "It is a powerful poison," he said, it takes at least ten days for its worst effects to clear away, and for its benefits to become clear. And, oh wow! His last day of radiation was the 13th! Incredible! It's been ten days! Why have we been so worried about Dad this week? Didn't he tell us that he would go downhill? This is a normal part of the healing process! We've been so stupid! We've been thinking the cancer was killing him, and all this time we've been seeing the natural action of his therapy, which Dad predicted! Maybe he didn't foresee dementia and trouble breathing, but, at a general level, everything is happening just exactly like he said it would! And tomorrow is day eleven! Tomorrow is the day that Dad begins to bounce back!!!

...

Later —

I definitely dozed off for a while. Dad is now feverish, hysterical, weak, writhing in pain. He is declining so fast now that one can see how much ground he has lost in just one night. In the cold light of day, the optimism of last night reveals itself as escapist fantasy—the kind of scenario we'd get if Hollywood was writing the script, the long-shot gamble that pays off, the unexpected happy ending that reunites the family in relative health just in time for Christmas. In real life, long shots rarely pay off.

...

My mom believes in the power of positive thinking. She has frequently said to me this year, "Dad is healing." My dad politely defers to her on this. I now wish I'd been more forceful in asking for the facts. Had I known how poorly my dad was doing, I might have begun looking for alternatives at an early date. Of course, I have only myself to blame for not

73

pressing the issue. But I'm not sure who I would have addressed my questions to. My mom regards positive thoughts as facts in themselves, and my dad, understandably, was holding onto the most positive interpretations of the information that the doctors gave him.

My dad dealt with 3 main doctors: one was in charge of his case in general, another was in charge of his radiation, and another was in charge of his chemo. I only learned this a few days ago, but apparently his main doctor was very blunt in his initial assessment back in March: cancer of the esophagus has one of the lowest survival rates, and my dad's chances were quite bad. The most optimistic of the doctors was the one in charge of the chemo. For months he would say such things as "This is a long shot, but there is a 1 in 100 chance this will work." (This, too, I only learned this week.)

Such language is misleading, even if it is factually accurate. Faced with death, people will cling to any treatment that gives them a chance, no matter how slim. until November, my folks seemed to quite honestly believe that my dad was going to make it. Certainly, until late November, they never communicated to me a bleak assessment of my dad's chances. I wish they had.

Most new drugs start off as research projects at universities. Researchers will pursue a lead that is buried in a mass of previously done work, then they will hone in on an active agent, and then begin double-blind tests on a test animal, such as a mouse or a monkey. If the results in the animals are both successful and safe, the researchers can move on to arranging tests on an appropriate human population. At this point, the university may enter into a royalty-sharing commercial agreement with a pharmaceutical company to help fund the research. It takes years to figure out how to get large amounts of the active ingredient, find the patients who can participate in the tests, clear the ethical and legal hurdles to using humans for research, and work out the royalty-sharing agreement with an interested corporation.

After all of that is arranged, the tests themselves can begin, and they often go on for years. If the human tests all go well, then (in the U.S.) the corporation can approach the FDA and begin the process of getting the drug legalized for commercial sale. The FDA may require additional tests for safety and effectiveness. This takes many more years. All of the new drugs that might become available to the general public in some future year, perhaps 2020, are being tested, right now, at universities across the world.

When I first learned my dad was sick, I planned to take some time off from work to investigate what the possibilities were. I am now angry at myself for not doing this sooner. If I have an excuse, it is that my dad had not yet exhausted traditional treatment options, and most experiments involving cancer drugs, because they are high risk, will only allow in patients who've already been declared terminal.

Last week I asked my dad about his parents and how they'd died. I'd already known that my grandmother died of breast cancer, but what I did not know was that she was fighting it for 6 years, from 1961 to 1967. Perhaps her experience influenced my dad's idea of how long he had to live. Perhaps he thought that even if he was going to die of cancer he might still have another 5 years.

...

December 24th. Later morning. My mom comes in. My dad is mumbling and unable to think clearly. The aide comes in and leaves his breakfast, but Dad is not able to eat. I make him tea, which he likes, with a lot of milk and some sugar. I'm trying to figure out ways to stop, or at least slow down, his loss of weight—and when he won't eat, giving him milk is a good option. It has protein. (My dad is down to 126 pounds now. He started the year around 190.)

I suspect Dad has a fever, so I go out to find the nurse. Unfortunately, the nurse on duty is Sandy, the worst of all the nurses. She is at her cart, filling out paperwork, checking charts, and taking medications in to her patients.

"Excuse me, nurse Sandy?" I say.

"Yes?"

"Could you come check on my dad? I think he might have a temperature."

She gives me a cool look, like she'd wish I'd just go away

and cease to exist.

"I'll be in in a few minutes," she mumbles.

Perhaps ten minutes later, she comes in and checks his temperature.

"He is at 99.9," she says. "That's borderline."

"Will you give him some Tylenol?" I ask.

"No. You've got to save that Tylenol. It can be hard on the liver. You only give it when someone has a real fever."

I'm certain that in my dad's delicate state, even low-grade fevers are contributing to his disorientation. But Sandy never compromises or negotiates with patients or their families.

"Can we watch his temperature carefully this morning?" I ask.

She hesitates for a moment, trying to figure out the most acceptable way to blow me off.

"I can check back later in the morning," she says.

I regard it as my responsibility to watch out for my dad's interests. I've sometimes been accused of not being aggressive enough when negotiating deals with my clients, and that is not a mistake that I want to make with my dad. I know that later, looking back, I'll feel better about myself if I err on the side of being too pushy with the medical staff, rather than not pushy enough. So I wait just 30 minutes before I go out into the hall and find Sandy again.

"Nurse Sandy?" I use the most placating, pleading voice that I can. I smile and try to look non-frantic. "Can you please check my dad's temperature again?"

She is at her cart staring at some kind of chart before her. She doesn't look at me. She tries to think of a way of blowing me off, but she be unable to think of an acceptable excuse, so she heaves a big sigh and then says, "Okay, I'll be in in a few minutes."

She comes in a few minutes later and takes my dad's temperature. It is now 100.9.

"Okay, now we can give Tylenol," she says.

My dad is nodding in and out, groggy, never fully awake. When we wake him, he's not talking, but he seems to understand us.

"Take this pill, Dad."

He takes it and washes it down with tea. Then he closes his eyes.

We wait.

...

It is 45 minutes since Dad took the Tylenol. His fever has come down. He has a lucid moment. He opens his eyes and looks at me.

"Hi, bearcub," he says. This is what he has called me since I was a child.

"Hi, Dad," I say.

"Hi, honeybear," says my mom.

"Hi, sweetie," he says.

His voice is very weak. His arms shake. He is in obvious discomfort, of the kind that seems to involve his whole body.

My mom starts to read off headlines from The New York Times. My dad basically says that he's lost all interest in politics because it no longer applies to him, but my mom seems to think that the headlines will distract him from his immediate problems. She did this to me when I was extremely sick, back in 1995, and it always drove me crazy.

He stares at my mom for a moment, then he turns and looks at me. There is a tear running down his cheek. Then he looks back at her.

"Kill me?" he says.

She looks up at him.

"Please?" he says.

Mom looks down and then looks at The New York Times. "You're not going to believe this article about J. Edgar Hoover," she says. "They say he had a plan to arrest 12,000 U.S. citizens during the Korean War. And he wanted to suspend habeas corpus."

"Please, honey," he says.

"Darling, you're healing, let's give you time to heal."

He rolls his eyes with frustration and looks up at the ceiling.

I have started to cry again and go over and take his hand.

"I love you, Dad," I say.

He opens his eyes again and looks at me.

"I love you, Lawrence."

"Are you in pain?" I ask.

He nods.

"I'll go get the nurse," I say.

He closes his eyes. I kiss him on the forehead and go out to find the nurse to ask her for more pain medication. The nurse says my dad is not eligible for more painkillers for an hour, so instead my mom and I roll him back and forth in the bed, a trick which sometimes relieves a little of the pain. But nothing can relieve his pain this morning.

An hour later, the nurse comes in and gives him more pain medication. He begins to drift off to sleep.

Now I feel I've done all that a good buddy can do. I am desperate to get some sleep. I kiss him goodbye, kiss my mother goodbye, tell them both that I love them, and leave. I drive back to my parents' home and get some sleep.

...

I arrive again at the rehabilitation clinic / medical center around 5 P.M. To my surprise, my brother Lance is here. My mom is watching the television. They have CNN on. My dad looks up at me. He lifts his arm, which is shaking with weakness, and he wriggles his fingers to say hello.

"Hello, Lawrence," he says.

"Hello, Dad."

I go over and give him a kiss. I am surprised that he is lucid; I thought perhaps we'd seen the last of his lucid periods.

I assume that Mom turned on the TV.

"Do we really need this?" I ask her.

Lance knows exactly why I'm asking, so he intercedes.

"No, no, no, Dad really did ask for this," he says.

My mom, with shocked innocence, says to me, "Darling, your father wanted to watch the news."

I look at Dad.

"Really, Dad? You want to watch the news?"

He nods. I am happy to sit down next to him and watch the news. I'm thinking this will be the last time we ever watch the news together.

The CNN debate for Democratic [presidential] nominees comes on. This is some sort of special debate with a focus on faith. All the questions are related to religion. I think it is ironic that this should be the last news show that an atheist like my father should watch. I think it must be a bitter pill for him to have lived through the high hopes of the 20th century, the rapid progress and modernization, and to have believed, for most of his life, that the U.S. was heading in a secular direction—and then, at the end of his life, to have the government taken over by right-wing Christian zealots and to have the national dialogue swamped with never-ending talk of God. All the same, we watch the show, and the candidates each comport themselves rather well.

"I wish Edwards was doing better in the polls," says my dad. Edwards, more than the other candidates, has focused on the level of income inequality in the country, and its effects. My dad feels this is the most crucial issue facing the country, and for that reason, he planned to vote for Edwards. But he knows now he will not live to see voting day.

A commercial comes on the television. It's for the Jenny Craig diet regime. An attractive actress, perhaps 30 years old, looks straight at the camera and smiles. "Last year I had a baby," she says, "and I gained a lot of weight." She puts her hands in front of her to indicate what a huge belly she once had. Right now she is looking somewhere between thin and average weight. "But with Jenny Craig, I was able to lose those excess pounds!" Now the camera cuts to some shots of delicious meals, lovely combinations of meats, cheeses, gravies and vegetables. A male voice announces the nutritional and tasty qualities of each dish and summarizes the cost of the Jenny Craig program. Then the camera cuts back to the female model. She smiles, spreads her arms widely and shouts, "I got my body back!"

Then the screen goes dark and the logo for CNN comes up. The camera cuts back to the news anchor, who begins a recap of today's top stories.

My dad, in a weak voice, says, "I wish I could get my body back."

...

I am determined that Dad will get his pain medication every three hours. In the past, the nurses have sometimes been as much as 45 minutes late, but I will not let that happen tonight. I want to be a good buddy for my dad. I must protect him from pain. I start to check the clock frequently. It is 9:10 P.M.; his next dose is at 9:30. I don't understand why this medical center is rationing the medication so strictly. He is going to be dead soon, so why not just hook him up to a permanent source of pain medication? Perhaps there are some legal implications? They need to protect him from overdosing? I will have to ask in the morning.

...

It is 10:57 P.M. My dad wakes up. He is holding his chest with both hands, and he is in great distress. He looks over at me.

"Get me up!"

"Where do you want to go, Dad?"

"Please!"

"What's the matter?"

"I can't breathe!"

"Okay, I'll go get the nurse."

I go out to the nurse's station. Maricel is just coming on duty.

"Excuse me," I say. I smile and try to appear non-frantic. "My dad is complaining of shortness of breath, and he seems to be in distress."

"Okay, I have two more patients and then I'll be in."

I go back inside the room.

"The nurse will be here soon, Dad."

"Please!"

"She's coming, Dad."

"Please."

"Hold my hand, Dad."

"I'm suffocating!"

"She's just out in the hallway, Dad."

"I'm dying!"

"Dad, I'm so sorry."

"Please!"

"Dad..."

"Help!"

I'm not sure what to say.

He turns toward the door.

"Help!" he yells as best he can. His voice is weak. He is hoping someone in the hallway can hear him.

I'm uncertain what to say.

"Help!" he yells again, with his weak voice.

"Let me check on the nurse," I say.

I go back into the hallway. The nurse is standing by her cart, filling out her paperwork. I walk up to her. She looks up at me. I smile and again try to appear non-frantic.

"My dad seems to be in a lot of distress," I say.

She, of course, already knows this, because I've already told her. I suppose at moments like this when I call upon the staff repeatedly that they begin to find me a pest. Maricel, however, is always professional, and doesn't ever allow herself to show a trace of annoyance. She smiles at me.

"I'll be right in," she says.

I go back in. My dad is still weakly shouting: "Help! Please! Help!"

He is holding his chest with both hands. I'm unsure if he is at the beginning of a heart attack.

"Okay, Dad, she is coming right in."

"Lawrence, please! Help!"

"I'm so sorry, Dad. I'm really so sorry."

"Lawrence!"

"She's coming soon, Dad."

"Hurry!"

His voice is getting weaker. I assume he's used up his oxygen. I hold his hand.

"Please!" he says. His voice is now a whisper.

The nurse comes in.

"How are you, Ralph?" she asks.

"Help?" my dad says. His voice is weak. His eyes are pleading with her.

"You're having shortness of breath?" she asks.

He nods. His voice is used up.

She puts the Pulsox on Dad's finger. Sure enough, his oxygen level has crashed to 81. It's the lowest oxygen number I've ever seen for him. Maricel is thoughtful.

"Help..." he says to her.

"We can put him on an oxygen tank for a while," she says.

She goes out, calls for some aides, then disappears down the hallway. I hold my dad's hand. Maricel and two aides come in with an oxygen tank. Since it is made of metal, I'm assuming that it can hold pressurized oxygen. The machine he's on currently simply delivers oxygen to his nose, with no pressure. Also, this tank comes with a full mask, which covers Dad's nose and mouth. The other machine simply delivered a tiny trickle of oxygen to his nose.

"I'm dying," he says.

"No, Ralph," says Maricel. "You'll feel the effect of this soon."

The mask is over Dad's face and the oxygen is being blown into his mouth and nose with some pressure.

Dad looks at me. "I'm suffocating," he says.

"This is going to help, Dad."

Maricel takes his pulse and waits. The Pulsox is on his finger. We're watching the numbers. They start to climb: 83, 84, 85.

"Just rest for a while, Ralph," says Maricel.

My dad stares at the wall in front of him. He looks beyond

despair. Maricel waits another few minutes and the numbers continue to go up.

"We cannot leave you on this tank all night," says Maricel. "So I'll be back in a little while."

Then she leaves.

Dad breathes in and out. He looks up at me. He blinks a few times. He is having trouble focusing.

"Lawrence?"

"Yes, Dad?"

"I'm so miserable."

"I'm so sorry, Dad. I'm so sorry. I'd do anything in the world for you that I could."

"I'm so miserable."

I hold his hand and he begins to doze off. Maricel comes back a half hour later and checks his oxygen again. It has gone up to 89.

"Good," she says. She disconnects him from the oxygen tank and puts him back on the other device.

"What are you doing?" he asks.

"Your oxygen is back up," she says. "So we can put you back on the other machine."

"Why?" I ask.

"He doesn't need the tank anymore," she says.

I'd ask more questions but I assume I won't get an answer that makes sense to me. I'm pleased that Dad seems more comfortable.

Maricel leaves and I stay right next to Dad's bed. He

stares at me for a little while, then at the wall in front of him, then he dozes off. I watch him as he sleeps. I wish, as before, that he could have a few more months with us, that we could talk about things, that we could review the good times and the bad; my childhood; talk about the way he remembers things and the way I remember things and the many things that we had shared together. Failing that, if he must go, I wish that he could go without pain.

I check the time again. It is 12:07 AM, the 25th of December, the beginning of Christmas morning. I wonder what Santa will bring us.

Subject: *the wrong way to die*
Date: *December 30, 2007*

I am very sad to say that my dad died this week. He died at 10:50 P.M. on the 26th of December. I have lost one of the greatest friends that I will ever have. His kindness, humor, intelligence, and open-mindedness were all things that I loved about him, and they are things I will greatly miss.

His death, I'm sad to say, was not pleasant—and watching him, and watching the staff at the facility where he died, I feel like I've learned a great deal about the medical system.

Despite a mix of Roxanol and Xanax (to calm him), my dad was largely unable to sleep during the early hours of the 25th. He was in too much pain. Over and over again he begged me to get help, and over and over again I went back out to the nurses to ask for help. The nurses, understandably, began to draw away from me. In contrast to earlier in the week, when they'd been quite helpful, now, when they saw me coming, they'd look away and try not to make eye contact; they would instead focus on the paperwork they were doing. When I got their attention, they politely explained that my dad already had all the painkillers he was allowed, and so there wasn't much they could do. I would go back to see my dad, who was bad by this point, and that would force me to go back and plead with the nurses. They would then come into the room and try to help in some physical way, for instance, rolling him from side to side sometimes helped to relieve the pressure in his spine. We'd also move around the pillows quite a bit, trying to make him more comfortable.

I recorded every conversation I had with my dad during the last week of his life. When I listen to the audio files, what I mostly hear, hour after hour, is his begging for help with the pain.

My dad was on enough medication that he often dozed off, but he did not sleep for more than 5 minutes before he would wake and again beg for relief from the pain. I kept hoping he might slip into a deep sleep, as he had on previous nights, but that didn't happen on this night. When the pain got very bad, and my dad was especially lucid, he would beg for death, hoping to escape the pain. When he was less lucid, a panic would come over him, and he would beg for his life. But, of course, there was nothing anyone could do to save his life.

Perhaps the hardest thing about the delirium is the way he would slip into a world where he irrationally thought he still had some hope of surviving, if only some nameless thing could be done, if only he could run away, if only he could hide from the dark forces that were coming after him.

My dad's delirium also undermined the treatment he got. At a very crucial moment, after he'd been begging me for help, I ran out and got the nurse to come in to see him. When the nurse and I came back into the room, he had dozed off. The nurse gently nudged him and he woke up disoriented. And she asked if he was in any pain. He said "No," which gave her some assurance that everything was okay. We moved some pillows around to make him comfortable. Then she left. Within 15 minutes, he was again begging me for help with his pain.

The worst of all the staff reactions was from Sandy, who seems to have decided that we (my family) were all somewhat hysterical. On the morning of the 25th, when she came on duty, my dad was still in great pain, and I went out to tell her this. She said that what I was seeing was a natural part of the process, and that the best "we" (she meant both the staff and my family) could do was to keep him "comfortable."

There were moments during this night when I felt like I was in some kind of insane asylum, but I could not figure out if I was the crazy one or if the staff was all crazy. In particular, whenever the staff told me that the goal was to keep my dad "comfortable," I had to wonder what the real meaning of the word was. The plain English meaning of the word wouldn't cover what I had seen all night, so I was left to question whether this was some sort of euphemism that medical professionals used to say, like, "There isn't much we can do."

Not knowing what else to do, I said to Sandy, "I'm not sure I know what the word 'comfortable' means."

With obvious irritation, she said, "You don't know what the word 'comfortable' means?"

"Well, I guess I was thinking that maybe we could do something about my dad's pain. He's been in pain all night."

With frustration, she said, "He's not in any pain! He's

having anxiety! That is what the Xanax is for!"

This conversation, more than most, motivated me to talk to the head nurse about potentially moving Dad to a hospital.

I was confused about many things all through this week. Why couldn't they just sedate my dad so that he could remain unconscious? Since he was going to die, why was it so important that he remain awake and alert? Was there really no way to get the pain under control? Why is it that when the government executes a criminal they first knock the criminal unconscious, but my dad was unable to get the same treatment? Also, why did he often have to take these drugs as a pill? Roxanol is a liquid form of morphine, why not simply give him large doses of that? He was having more and more trouble coming out of his delirium long enough to recognize what a pill was. Swallowing was difficult for him. What were they going to do when he fell unconscious? How would they get him pain-killing medication at that point?

As the night wore on, I became convinced that we had made a terrible mistake by keeping my dad at the rehab center. We had to get him to a hospital. As soon as my mom came in at 8 AM, she and I asked for a meeting with the head nurse. We were going to propose moving him to a hospital.

However, at this point everything changed. A new head nurse came on duty, a lovely woman from Russia named Yulena, and her attitude was quite different than what I'd encountered all night long. Perhaps it was because we were threatening to go to a hospital, which maybe would have reflected poorly on her institution. I'll never really know.

She called Dr. Patel immediately, and he authorized a huge increase in the pain medication that my dad was receiving. Dad's dose of Roxanol was more than doubled, and he was put on Fentanyl, too. Best of all, his medications were now all liquid, so he no longer had to take pills. If he fell unconscious, it would be enough to squirt the Roxanol into his mouth, where it would get absorbed through the skin. The Fentanyl was in a patch that attached to his skin on his inner arm, and the patch slowly released a steady stream of painkillers into his system.

This new regimen finally got dad's pain mostly under control. I feel terrible that I wasn't more aggressive with the staff during the night—he suffered hours of horrific, agonizing pain. Everything that was done in the morning should have been done the previous night. I wanted to be a good buddy to him, but I think I let him down. I had promised to defend him from pain, and then I let him die a horrible, agonizing death. For a substantial period of the last 4 days of his life, he was under-medicated.

Out of that awful, confusing night, I am certain of only one thing: This was not what my dad wanted, and had he known of the horrific levels of pain that he was going to have to endure, he never would have consented to die at this place.

With his pain under control, my dad fell asleep, and then I went home and got some sleep.

I returned in the evening, around 6 P.M. I was somewhat

surprised that he was awake and lucid. He was also fairly comfortable, the pain medication finally being adequate.

My aunt Miriam (my mom's sister) and Uncle Irving were visiting. Dad had been asleep when they first showed up, but now we all went into his room together and he was awake.

"Hi, Irv," said my dad. He said this in a cheerful, friendly way. I found this endearing, because it was so normal, and it reminded me of how sweet and good-natured he was when he was not in pain.

Aunt Miriam went off on a long riff about all the toys that various grandchildren had just gotten that day for Christmas. She was good about holding the floor and providing entertainment. She knew how to package events into neat, funny anecdotes. Dad did very little talking; he mostly just listened.

Later, Mom and Aunt Miriam and Uncle Irving were standing in the corner of the room, and then my aunt and uncle put their coats on and started to go out. My dad wasn't clear why they were leaving without saying goodbye, but in a very cheerful, friendly voice, he said, "Goodbye, everybody!"

Apparently they'd all thought he was asleep. They went back over to him and said their goodbyes. Then they went out. A while later, Mom also left.

These goodbyes were the last conversations where my dad was lucid, so they remain precious to me.

After everyone left, I asked Dad if he was thirsty and he said yes. I got him some tea and milk, and he took a few sips. This was to be the last drink he ever had. After that he fell asleep.

The early hours of the 26th were horrifying, but not the way the early hours of the 25th had been. My dad slept most of the night. Only a few times did he wake up and try to get out of bed. The panic was pressing in close on him now, the sense that death was near and he had to escape. He was weaker now than I'd ever seen him. Sometimes, without even opening his eyes, he would reach out into the air with his hands and grasp at things that were not there. I've no idea what kind of nightmares or hallucinations were haunting him.

He was, more and more, unable to talk because of the lack of oxygen. When he woke, he would hold his hands to his chest to indicate that he felt he was suffocating. When the nurse came in to check his blood oxygen level, I found that I no longer had the courage to look and see what the number was. My dad was dying. There was nothing I could do except cry. I cried most of the night, almost every time I looked at him.

He was unconscious for a long time. Every previous night, a big part of my job had been getting him liquids. Now he went the whole night without liquids. The few times he woke up, I tried to get him to take a sip of water, which I would ready for him on a small plastic spoon. During the night, he took no more than 3 small half-filled spoons of water. Most of the time, in his panic, he pushed me away. It's possible that, in his hallucinations, he began to perceive me as one of the dark forces trying to hurt him.

Toward dawn, a nurse came in and I asked if there was anything I could do to provide moisture for my dad. She got me some swabs that could absorb water. She told me I could use them to keep his lips moist, and if I put them in his mouth, sometimes the gag reflex would cause a person to close their mouth and suck on them. I used one in my own mouth to get a sense for how it felt and how far back I could go before triggering serious gagging. I used it on my dad. He never clamped down on it, but I'd like to think I helped to keep his mouth moist.

My mom came in at 8 A.M. My dad woke up and had a terrifying episode He was frantic about the lack of oxygen. He could no longer talk. Nurse Sandy suggested Xanax, to help with the panic. She mashed it up into apple sauce, and my mom got him to put it in his mouth. I waited for it to take effect. Some time after that, he became unconscious. He never regained consciousness.

During the last 36 hours of my dad's life, it got harder and harder to figure out what being a "good buddy" really meant. I knew he was suffering from lack of oxygen. I asked the nurses about giving him an oxygen tank again. All of them asked the same question: "Is he DNR?" He is. That seems to mean there is no point helping him past a certain point. Something must fail. Maybe it'll be his lungs, or his kidneys, or his heart, but something must fail, and it will be horrible when it does, and he will suffer. This was very hard to accept, and very hard to watch.

I got back to the medical center at 6 P.M. on the 26th. I relieved mom, who'd been with Dad all day. I sat and watched him. He was unconscious now, but his eyes were open. He wasn't blinking. After a while it occurred to me that his eyes must be very dry. I mentioned this on the phone to my friend Wendy, a former nurse, and she suggested that I close his eyes. I tried to, but his eyes wouldn't close. She said that likely his cornea had dried out, so she suggested I go get saline solution from the staff and water his eyes. I went and did this, and I kept Dad's eyes moist until he was dead. This was, of course, a totally futile effort at making him comfortable, but until the end, I wanted to do what little I could.

Over and over again, we expected the medical staff to educate us about what our options were, whereas they expected us to educate ourselves. To give an example, on the evening of the 26th, when I got back to the medical center, I asked my mom if Dad had had any liquids all day, and she said no.

While it was obvious that he was about to die, somehow it seemed very sad to me that he should die of dehydration. For some reason, that struck me as an especially horrible way to die. So my mom and I approached the head nurse to ask her about this. Her first question, of course, was whether he was DNR, and we said yes and then we felt silly. She, no doubt, thought the whole conversation was silly, too, since he was DNR, so taking measures once he was unconscious seemed pointless to her. She was too polite to say this, of course. Instead, sensing that we wanted to see my dad cared for, she asked us if he was "hospice." We didn't know what that was, so we asked. She explained that it meant a higher level of care: a nurse that would come in for an hour each day and look after him. Mind you, we were being told of this option exactly 3 hours and 20 minutes before he died. Had someone mentioned it to us a week before, or a month before, we would have opted for it.

Another surprise for me is what happened once my dad actually died. I watched as he took his final breath, then the nurse came in, then she got the head nurse, and then they made the official pronouncement. They left me alone with him for a while, and then I made some phone calls, and then I went home and got my mom.

After we'd returned to the rehab center, we both said our goodbyes to Dad. After that, we asked nurse Maricel what happened next. She asked us how we were going to get the body out of there. We were shocked by that; we assumed they had some way of handling the body. Maricel was shocked by our shock.

"Uh, you have no way of handling this body tonight?" asked Maricel.

My mom said, "Can we leave it here tonight and figure out what to do with it in the morning?"

Maricel was too professional to curse, but her facial expression said, "What the hell am I going to do with this body?" She then looked around the room, trying to come up with a plan. Aloud, she said, "Maybe if we make it very cold in here?"

She looked at the window and tried to calculate whether it would be cold enough if she turned the heat off and left the window open. As it was December in New Jersey, it was very cold outside.

This was another situation where we had assumed the staff would educate us about what to do, whereas they had assumed we would educate ourselves. Given time, we probably would have, but even one week before, we'd still been thinking that dad might live a few more months, and the speed at which his illness moved had caught us off-guard.

"I'll need to check with my supervisor about what to do," said Maricel. Then she went out. We were left with my dad. I sat with him a long time. Neither my mom nor I could stop crying.

It was about 2 A.M. by the time Maricel came back and said that they could not keep the body until morning. We had to find a funeral home to come and pick it up. My mom and I went out to the nurse's desk and they gave us a phone book. My mom looked through the yellow pages and called several places. Then she remembered one place that she'd dealt with a long time ago, a place where she'd had a positive experience, so she called them and made arrangements. They said they would send someone out within an hour.

All in all, it was a confusing week, full of horror.

As to the right way to die, I'm left with the impression

that if a person has a terminal illness, the best way to die is probably at home, after taking a lethal amount of painkillers. It needs to be done carefully, of course, but I'm guessing this might be the best way. This is probably what I would prefer, if I were sure that I was terminal and had no treatment options left.

The tendency, I suspect, would be to put off the final moment for as long as possible, although, as my dad's case demonstrates, the longer one delays, the more chance there is that something will happen which will render a person unable to follow this course.

The second best way to die, if a person has the health insurance to pay for it, is probably in a well-staffed hospital, where the nurses can stay on top of one's situation as one goes downhill. I assume that in a place with a lot of nurses, it is easier to ensure that a dying person always has a sufficient amount of painkillers. A medical center of the type we dealt with doesn't have enough nurses (one nurse for every 16 patients) to handle a real crisis situation like what my dad faced. All the same, such medical centers represent the future, as both hospitals and insurance companies are promoting them due to their low cost. So it is likely that more and more people are going to die in such institutions.

As for my dad, I am heartbroken that he is gone. I have trouble imagining there will ever be a time when I don't miss him.

Part II

Regarding My Mom's Illness

A dream: Dad and I are cleaning the family house in Jackson, New Jersey. Mom comes into the room and tells us not to throw away any of her magazines. Dad and I look at each other and roll our eyes. Mom and her magazines! We have so many magazines! It's crazy. But okay. We share a moment of humor. My girlfriend is driving to the restaurant, we should get in the car and drive to meet her. Mom says, "Okay, I'll get my coat." An odd thought occurs to me: Wasn't there a moment in the past when my dad died? And yet here he is, right next to me. I look at his hair, his eyes; I listen to his voice. This is definitely Dad. He is definitely alive. And yet I have a memory of him dying. How is that possible?

Then I wake up.

More than twelve years have passed and yet I still dream of my father almost every night. He is always in my thoughts. The pain has never abated. I imagine I'll go to my grave still grieving.

Getting through 2008 was especially difficult, for me and for my mother. She continued with her political work with the Environmental Commission and the League of Women Voters. She also became much more active with her church, which on Thursdays ran a book club. I think this operated a bit like group therapy for her.

Time passed. The sorrow remained. Still, my mom soldiered on with remarkable courage and vitality. Our town of Jackson continued to hold her in high regard, thanks to her work with the city government. But no one can remain young forever.

I never had to worry about my parents so long as the two of them were alive and healthy, but once my mom was living alone, I found that I was often concerned about her. In 2009, I moved from Virginia to New York City. Partly that was for my career, but it was also planned so I could keep a closer eye on her. During the first few years, she was still healthy. She traveled often—to see a friend in Canada, to see my brother out in San Francisco. Still, I would go visit with her twice a month, to say hello and to help fix things around the house when she needed such help.

A healthy adult is Okay. When you are in the main part of life, that does not seem like a big deal. As we get older, hanging onto that status becomes important. My mom fought hard to maintain the life of an Okay adult. That meant pretending she was still strong, alert, and self-sufficient. After a certain point, it was stressful, for me and I think also for her, to go on pretending that she was still at the Okay part of her life. Eventually, there arrived a crisis that forced us to acknowledge that she was Not Okay. Recognizing that she was weakening meant recognizing her mortality, and that was a very painful reckoning. And yet, there was a certain relief, when the day finally came, in that we no longer had to go on pretending that she was still an Okay adult.

By 2017, my mom's driving was a little bit erratic. I suggested she start thinking about the end of an era; she got angry and argued that she was a great driver. At some point I decided I no longer wanted to see her driving. I wasn't able to convince her that major changes might be coming to her life, so I began to spend most of the week at her house so I could drive her where she wanted to go. As I write software and develop software systems architecture for a living, I'm lucky that I can often work remotely and make my own schedule.

Towards the end of 2018, my mom developed a cough. It was a startling development, because she had (no exaggeration) never had a cough before. Her immune system was legendary; she simply never got sick. For instance in 1993, at the end of her teaching career, she was allowed to cash in her unused sick days. Turns out that she received a nice chunk of change, since she had accrued an astonishing 190 unused sick days. Because of her unusually invincible health (and a large dose of pure stubbornness), she had managed to arrive at her 90th birthday without ever having acquired a family doctor. Most people her age see a doctor on a regular basis but my mom had gone decades without seeing one.

By the middle of December 2018, I was very worried. I repeatedly urged my mom to find a doctor who could listen to her lungs. My mom refused. She took more vitamins. She was sure she would bounce back. Again, she had almost no experience with illness, so I initially understood how novel this might have been for her.

By January 1st, she was in really bad shape. She was running a fever and she seemed weaker than normal. Since our religious beliefs are different, she almost never asked me to pray with her, but now she did. She seemed to realize that she needed help, but she was still too stubborn to go see a doctor.

We went for a walk. She fell. She was hurt.

This set in motion eight intense weeks during which I was constantly interacting with medical establishments. These interactions were as frustrating as my experiences twelve years before, but they were frustrating to me in different ways. Once again, I was confronted with the weaknesses in the U.S. health system and how that system communicates with people who typically show up at a hospital during their worst moments when we're afraid, under a great deal of stress, and we generally fail to think clearly enough to ask the questions we really need to ask.

As before, I recorded these events mostly by writing email to my friends. I'd like to share some of these emails so you can see the mistakes I made and hopefully avoid them yourself.

Subject: *a fall happens in less than one second, and the injury can change one's entire life*

Date: *January 6, 2019*

Dear Ewelina,

Back in 1979, my mom had what seemed like a bad fall. She was coming down the stairs at our house. I think she was carrying some laundry. She lost her grip on the laundry basket, which slipped down to her feet and then tripped her. She then fell down the rest of the stairs, about 6 steps. She landed at the bottom. I was at the front door, so I saw the whole thing. Surprisingly, she was unhurt. She sat there, stunned, for a moment. We all rushed to help her. She sat there and she said a prayer out loud. Then she got back up and she was fine. No injuries.

I was only 12 years old back then. I'm glad she wasn't hurt. And I'm glad she's enjoyed another 40 healthy years.

These last few weeks, she's had a cough. It's slowly gotten worse. I suggested she see a doctor and she refused. I suggested that she take some of my antibiotics and she refused. I was worried about her cough turning into pneumonia. She was having trouble sleeping. I felt her forehead and she felt hot. I told her she might have a fever. She told me I was being ridiculous.

On Wednesday, she went upstairs to her office to check her email. I was in the dining room, working for a client. Around 3:30 P.M., she told me she wanted to go out for a walk.

This sent up a red flag for me. She absolutely hates the cold. "Mom, are you okay?"

Abruptly, she snapped at me. "Of course I'm okay!"

I checked her forehead again; she felt warm. I was certain she had a fever.

I reluctantly began helping her put her coat on. My better judgment wanted to tell her to stay inside, but I also knew that such a request would've been completely futile. My mother is an extremely strong, independent woman. Actually that's putting it lightly.

I touched the sleeve of her coat and posed the question again. "Mom, listen to me. Are you okay?"

With the same anger she responded, "I just said I'm okay!"

We went out. Only wide enough for one person, the sidewalk didn't allow us to walk side by side—so I gave it to her, while I walked along in the street. I didn't want to expose my mom to the danger of walking in the street, though it had been newly paved, so in that sense it was safer than the sidewalk, which was badly cracked. We were chatting about the Democrats taking over the House of Representatives, and how this would make life difficult for President Trump.

A car came up the street. I glanced at it for safety's sake. It gave me a wide berth.

I looked back at my mom. She was lying flat on the ground. I had only looked away for 1 second, yet everything had changed.

She was not moving. For a split second I thought that she would surely get up, and we would laugh about this, perhaps go back to the house, check if she were hurt. But my heart began to accelerate and the pressure built in my arteries as my body reacted the same speed as my mind. Something was very wrong.

"Mom?" I asked.

No response. She lay facedown, without any movement.

I knelt down and tried to turn her over. She felt very heavy.

"Mom?" I asked. "Mom?"

She didn't respond at all. I thought she might be dead.

I put both of my arms around her completely and pulled her onto my lap. Now her eyes opened.

"Lawrence?" she asked. She was dazed. Blood was coming down from her forehead.

I tried to stand up with her and realized I couldn't. I felt I had to get her back to the house, and then we would call 911. We were only 100 meters from home. I wasn't sure how to get her back. Without at least some degree of effort on her part, she was too solid to easily get up off the ground.

"Help!" I shouted. "Help! Help!"

I was screaming at the top of my lungs. I had no clear plan, only the sense that something was very wrong. It seemed almost certain that we needed to go to the hospital, though I wanted her to be revived enough to realize this herself and then agree with me. Although she had a bad cut on her head, and the blood was coming down over her right eye, she wasn't bleeding at such a rate that we needed to immediately cauterize the injury. If we could get home, we could take a few minutes to collect whatever might be important before we headed to the hospital. She would need her pocketbook, her health insurance card, and her ID, and perhaps a change of clothes. I could see the house from where we sat on the sidewalk; it was simply a question of whether I'd be able to get her there.

We were in front of a neighbor's property. A person in the house briefly opened the curtain, looked at us, then closed the curtain. I shouted "Help!" as loudly I could. They certainly heard me. They were 10 meters away and I was screaming as loud as I could. They hid within their house. Perhaps they were worried about lawsuits. Legally, in New Jersey, each home owner is responsible for maintaining the safety of the sidewalk in front of their house. I recall my dad worrying about that (even though any lawsuit would be paid by the homeowner's insurance). But nowadays, nobody really seems to worry about it. There are cracked and uneven sidewalks throughout the neighborhood.

Two boys, both in their early teens, came along the street on bicycles. The first, a bit overweight, squinted at us as if he couldn't understand what he was seeing. They slowed to the point that they were hardly moving and gaped at us without offering to help.

"Hey!" I said. "Can you help me get my mom up? She's

fallen."

"Hey, mister," said the heavy one. "You need to go to the hospital."

"Can you help us stand up?" I asked.

The other boy looked intensely uncomfortable but said nothing. The first boy repeated himself again: "You need to go to the hospital."

They slowed down, but they never stopped. It's possible they were frightened and didn't want to get involved.

"Can you please help us?" I asked again.

"Mister," said the first boy. "What are you doing? Go to a hospital." By then, they had passed us. They picked up their pace and quickly disappeared around a corner.

Life is an improvisational act, always, but especially during a crisis, when we are forced to plainly see the provisional nature of our everyday life. Above all else, a crisis is when we notice our audience, the fear on their faces, the curiosity, the disgust. And every person we've ever known is, in part, a member of the audience, observing our performance. In good moments, we enjoy the interaction, and our performance is shaped by the audience response. But when things are bleak, failing to pull the crowd along with us is a terrible feat.

"Lawrence?" asked my mom. "What happened?"

"You fell," I said. "Can you get up?"

"Okay," she said mechanically, still dazed. She didn't move.

"Can you get up?" I asked.

"Okay," she said again, but she did not move. I wondered if she was paralyzed.

A car stopped. A woman in her 50s got out.

"Did she fall?" asked the woman.

"Yes," I said. "Can you help me get her up?"

The woman took one of my mother's arms. Together, we got Mom to her feet. The woman had some tissues and pressed them to the gash on my mom's head.

"Have you called 911?" asked the woman.

"Not yet," I said.

At least that managed to get a reaction from my mom. She said, "Lawrence, please, no hospitals. Don't put me through that. Please? Don't call 911. I don't want to go to the hospital."

The woman told her, "You need to go to the hospital. You're bleeding very badly."

"Mom, we have to go to the hospital."

The woman said, "I'll call 911 for you."

"Thank you," I said. She asked me for my number, which I relayed to her and she relayed to Emergency Services.

My mom said, "Lawrence, I want to go home."

I asked, "Can you walk?"

"Of course," she said, but she was having trouble walking.

"Can you take a step?" I asked.

She took an awkward step. I still had my right arm around her and I was holding her up.

"Good, Mom. Good!" I said. "Can you take another step?"

She took another awkward step. It was slow going, but we were moving.

In the moment, I had no idea what was going on. The whole thing was a confusing series of events which I failed to understand. Only hours later, at the hospital, when a doctor asked if my mom had been knocked unconscious, did I first begin to consider the possibility. Her lack of any response, followed by her disorientation, would be consistent with a blow to the head so severe that she was actually unconscious for a moment.

We took another step, and then another step. We eventually reached the lawn of our house. By now she was coming back to herself.

Our good Samaritan, the woman from the car who'd stopped for us, stayed with us until we got to the door. I briefly thanked her. I'm sure she understood why I wasn't more loquacious when I wished her goodbye.

Mom went to the bathroom to see how bad it was. I think when she saw all the blood, she realized that she would indeed have to go to the hospital.

Only now, as I write these words, does the whole episode resolve itself into a story. Full sentences, full of words, obeying the rules of correct grammar, automatically become more coherent than a real-life emergency ever is. In the moment, my heart was racing, and my sense of what was happening to my mom was in rapid flux. Chaos is pre-verbal; panic lacks words. My point is, everything sounds more obvious now that I'm writing about it. But while events were unfolding, all I felt was confusion.

Very briefly, my mom pulled herself together, and again she asserted that she did not want to go to a hospital. She was holding a bandage to her head. Given the strength of her conviction, I had to wonder, what was prudent? How much should I bow to her picture of comfort, versus what was surely the safer course? I finally decided we absolutely had to go. This probably sounds like a complicated process, and yet in reality I spent only a few seconds considering all of the options.

"Mom, we must go," I said. "This is not optional. You have a fever. You are seriously injured. You might have a broken bone. We need to have someone check you and make sure you are okay."

She finally acquiesced, and we began to gather her things.

Emergency Services called me. They were annoyed because we weren't at the location from which the 911 call had been made. I explained we'd come back up the street and gave our address. As they were only half a block away, they arrived just a few seconds after I gave them the correct location.

Many hours later, I realized a minor change would have made my mom's fall much less serious. My mom's hands are very sensitive to cold. So she had had put on gloves and then stuck her gloved hands deep into the pockets of her big coat.

When she tripped, she couldn't put her hands out in front of her. So she fell directly onto her face. If she had simply had her hands free, then she would probably not have been as seriously hurt. Yet all the same, I'd been wanting a doctor to examine her because of the very dangerous cough that she had developed, and now we were going to a hospital.

For weeks I'd been asking my mom to see a doctor and for weeks she had been refusing. Despite the terrible circumstances, there was a silver lining, in the sense that her lungs would finally be examined.

We went to the Jersey Shore University Medical Center. We arrived at 5:00 P.M. The eye doctor came to see my mom at 10:00 P.M. He said the injury to her right eye was profound and recommended that we transfer to Rutgers University Hospital at Newark, which had a team of specialist eye surgeons. We agreed.

"It's important that you have this surgery within 24 hours of the injury," said the doctor.

I waited until midnight, but no transfer had come through. They told me it was scheduled for 3:00 A.M. I told my mom I would go home and get some sleep and then come see her as early as possible in the morning.

I got a phone call in the middle of the night that confirmed that she had been transferred.

I arrived at the hospital at Newark at 9:00 A.M. and was told she was still in the emergency room. I was angry about this. She had been waiting 6 hours in the emergency room! I went to the ER, but they had just transferred her upstairs. I went upstairs and found her room. She was glad to see me. I was glad to see her and also very sad.

Her cough was bad. They did a chest X-ray and decided she probably had pneumonia. This confirmed what I had been fearing for the previous two weeks.

I've read that in terms of surgery, to repair an eye injury, it's crucial that the surgery happen within the first 72 hours of the injury. So I initially thought they should prioritize this. But that was before I understood how serious my mom's pneumonia was.

It was crucial to have an eye specialist study my mom's eye, so eventually she was taken to see Dr. Zarbin. He struck me as very intelligent and methodical. He studied my mom's right eye for a long time and eventually formed a theory about what had happened: Since my mom had once had cataracts, there was a seam where her eye had been sewed shut after the cataract surgery. He now believed that when she fell, that seam had ruptured. So that would need to be sewn shut again. However, he warned, it would not be possible to restore normal sight in that eye. My mom might be able to again see light and dark, but she would not be able to use that eye to, for instance, read a newspaper. For all normal functions, she would be relying on her other eye for the rest of her life.

Nevertheless, surgery was scheduled for the next day. I stayed with my mom until midnight, then headed home for a few hours of sleep, then turned around and got back to the hospital not long after dawn.

I was told that my mom's pneumonia seemed to be getting worse. Despite an IV of antibiotics, her white blood cell count remained stubbornly high. Worse, the previous night, for the first time, her blood oxygen level dipped and they had to put her on an oxygen tank.

Yet they were going ahead with the surgery? How had that decision been made?

When I look back at my experience with my father, I feel that I didn't fight fiercely enough for him, I didn't ask enough questions, I didn't educate myself enough. I'd assumed the system would work for him. And in some important ways, the system had failed my family. This time, while my mom was in the hospital, I was determined to manage the situation more effectively than I had for my father. In particular, I was no longer assuming that any decision made by the doctors was automatically the right decision. It was up to us to ask hard questions and make sure the answers made sense.

Was it safe for my mom to undergo surgery when her pneumonia was out of control and she'd already suffered a low oxygen moment? Did it make sense to take such a risk when there was no hope of restoring perfect sight? If sight in that eye was going to be damaged for the rest of her life, no matter what we did, why should she face the trauma of serious surgery at a time when she was fighting for her life?

A crucial question for me was: Who was actually making that decision? And what I realized was that, in the most fundamental sense, no one was making the decision. The system was making the decision. Or rather, the decision was up to us. Essentially, we wouldn't get help from the medical professionals. As there were no perfect options, what we faced was a situation where we had to balance the risks of one choice against another choice. We could risk surgery on the off-chance she might regain perception of light and dark in the damaged eye, or we could skip the surgery and Mom could save her strength and use it to fight the pneumonia.

Over the years, my mom had functioned as editor for several books by a writer we knew in Charlottesville, VA. This woman was 10 years younger than my mom and had been in good health when she was crossing a street and an off-duty police officer barreled through the intersection without seeing her. Our writer friend ended up with a badly damaged knee and had to go for surgery. But something happened to her while she was in the care of the anesthesiologist. Although, in theory, the surgery had gone well, she had a fogginess of the mind afterward. She had written 20 books in the past, but she was never able to write again after her hospitalization. That clarity of mind for which she'd been known was gone forever. And she went for that surgery when she was otherwise in good health. Unlike my mom, she hadn't been fighting pneumonia. Her story weighed on us. We knew that even healthy people could suffer adverse consequences from surgery, and now my mom was very sick.

In all of our troubles, one of the blessings we enjoyed

was that my mom had a good relationship with the minister of her church, the Reverend Angela Denton, a truly lovely person and someone who radiated confidence (as people who are solid in their faith often are). Reverend Denton came to visit and spent most of the day with us. When we were taken to the surgery prep room, Reverend Denton came with us. For a long while we prayed together, asking for good fortune regarding my mom's health.

Way back in the 1970s, my mom had discovered the Unity Church, and she attended occasionally during those years. I'm uncertain what first drew her to it. At the risk of putting words into her mouth, I'll say it is an unusually open, tolerant, and accepting Church. Having grown up in a household full of all kinds of dogmatism, my mom was looking for a community that emphasized love rather than catechism.

After my father's death, Unity Church became especially important to my mom. She became an active member and was eventually elected to the Board, where she served as the treasurer for six years.

Diving deeper into her faith, my mom attended the Thursday book club that the Reverend organized each week. I have the impression that the book club drew the most interested members, eager to read interesting spiritual texts, and to discuss them with others who shared the same kind of intellectual and spiritual wonder. I also have the impression that, for my mom, the book club acted as a kind of group therapy session, and allowed her to process some of the grief she felt regarding the loss of my father. The Unity Church became an essential part of my mom's life, and gave her the strength to go on enjoying life, despite the devastation of her loss. Certainly, while my mom was in the hospital, the support of the church community was a wonderful psychological support.

As events unfolded, we were glad to have the Reverend come to the hospital to pray with us.

A medic came over and told us that we had 15 minutes left.

What should we do? My mom was opposed to the surgery, but I knew that she feared all surgery simply because she didn't trust doctors. I felt my own role had to be to get my mom to overcome her fear, if overcoming her fear was best for the long-term. But I wasn't convinced that surgery was a good idea. And I was deeply concerned that the medical professionals didn't have the same sense of trepidation that I had.

Finally, they came to get my mom. I had some questions. I asked the woman who was to lead the surgery: Are you not worried about the pneumonia? My mom has already suffered a low oxygen incident. The doctor looked puzzled and asked if anesthesiologist had given the okay. She went away to check with the nurses. She came back and told me that if the anesthesiologist was confident then she didn't feel comfortable second-guessing the decision. I asked her if we could wait a day and try to get the pneumonia under slightly better control. The woman called over the nurses, who then tried to call the doctor who was overseeing the treatment of my mom's lungs. They weren't able to reach that doctor. And it was time for the surgery. The room had been reserved for my mom, the team had been assembled, and it was important to maintain the schedule.

More than ever before, it felt like a decision was being made to offer maximum comfort to the logistical needs of the institution, rather than to offer maximum consideration of the unique circumstances of my mother. Because of the highly specialized nature of modern medicine, there was no one person who was responsible for her entire, unified health. Instead, each doctor had his or her specialty, and no doctor was willing to step on the toes of any other specialist.

One doctor saw my mother as a set of lungs, another doctor saw my mother as a heart and respiratory system to be kept going while paralyzed during surgery, another doctor saw my mother as an eyeball to be operated on. None saw her as my mother.

We asked for another moment. I requested that the minister lead us in a prayer during which we would ask God for clarity. After this, Reverend Denton had to leave us. We thanked her and said goodbye.

Only a few moments were left. My mom and I talked, trying to imagine the two paths before us. I came around to the view that we should cancel the surgery. The risks seemed high and the benefits seemed doubtful.

Hoping to shield my mom from the brunt of anyone's

anger, I made our joint decision known to the surgeon. They were, somewhat understandably, upset that we hadn't made the decision much sooner. They explained that they had been at a different hospital and had driven here just to take care of my mom. I apologized for our late decision. But our decision was final.

I should emphasize that defying an institution this late in the decision-making process is enormously stressful. If you ever find yourself in a similar situation, try to make your final decision sooner, or be prepared to stand up to a considerable amount of anger and griping.

Then the doctors started doing all of the necessary paperwork. This took almost an hour! It's amazing how slow hospitals can be. My mom and I went out to the hall and paced back and forth. Walking seemed to make my mom feel better, like she was still in control of things.

Finally, they sent a nurse with a wheelchair who took my mom back to her room.

Now the whole focus was on her pneumonia. They gave her massive amounts of antibiotics through an IV. But the hours went by and it didn't seem to help. Right now, they're tracking her white blood cell count, which is very high. They're waiting for that to come down.

They're keeping her at the hospital at least until Tuesday. Once her cough is better, she can come home. I'll keep you posted.

Subject: *my mom's condition has improved*

Date: *January 7th, 2019*

Dear Misty,

Just an update. The doctors are using my mom's white blood cell count to track the severity of her pneumonia. Apparently that number has improved. So they're ready to release her from the hospital. They're also recommending physical rehabilitation. My mom has agreed to this. So at some point today or tomorrow she will be transferred to a rehab clinic. They suggest she stay there at least a week. Pneumonia is so terrible that it can make a healthy young person feel weak, and for someone like my mom, it has profoundly weakened her, so I think physical rehab is a good idea.

Subject: *slow improvement, which leaves us facing the next few steps*
Date: *January 9, 2019*

Dear Kristin,

Thank you for writing. I'm pleased to say that my mom is getting better. Her white blood cell count is coming down, which means the pneumonia is getting better. They will be releasing her from the hospital today, I hope. She will follow up with physical therapy.

We face a problem, though. My mom used to have very good health insurance. She was a teacher and the teachers have a strong labor union. Even retired teachers are supposed to have good health insurance. When my dad was sick in 2007, my mom's health insurance paid for excellent care. But then in 2010 the state of New Jersey elected Chris Christie, who is a Republican. He pushed through a law that decreased the level of health insurance for retirees. So my mom's health insurance is bad now, and it's difficult to find a rehabilitation clinic that will take her. The doctors authorized her release on Monday, yet now it is Wednesday and we are still here at the hospital, still hoping to find a place that will accept my mom's insurance.

Dear Kristin,

I hope you'll forgive me writing an email that is full of complaints, but every aspect of the U.S. health care system seems full of frustrations, almost as if it was designed to maximize the frustration.

After waiting many days for health insurance to give approval for my mom to get physical therapy, we were denied at every single clinic we applied to. I assume it's because they lacked beds or there was a problem with the insurance. I had asked that she be moved south so she would be closer to home, but instead, my mom's case worker lined us up with a clinic up north. It was the only place that would take Mom, I guess? This place is out in north Jersey. From New York, it takes me 90 minutes to get there, and from my mom's house it takes about 105 minutes.

The food is expensive, but not good. I felt bad for my mom when I saw her lunch; it is the simplest, most boring sandwich you can imagine, just some egg salad with 2 slices of bread. Not even a tomato. Not even lettuce.

At the hospital, I was told this clinic was very important because my mom would get 2 hours a day of intense physical therapy. But it's nothing like that. I was with her for the morning session. She was taken to the therapy room for 45 minutes, but most of the time she just sat there in her wheelchair.

She only interacted with the therapist for 15 minutes, some of which simply consisted of my mom being told to bend a rubber bar: "Bend that bar! Keep bending it!" The therapy room was crowded with patients and they each had to wait to get a few minutes of time with the therapist.

Two weeks ago, my mom and I went to the park near her house and we walked the Bracken Trail. That was 30 minutes of real exercise, which is twice as much as she got today, and we didn't have to spend thousands of dollars to do it.

Later on, my mom got a bit stir crazy, so we walked the halls. She can walk fine so long as she has something to lean on. She used her wheelchair as if it were a walker.

Meanwhile, she hasn't fully recovered from the pneumonia, but they switched her to oral antibiotics, and now her cough seems to be getting worse. But there are no doctors at the facility during the weekend, so I couldn't talk to anyone about the most urgent health issue she's facing. I'll have to makes some calls.

The whole thing made me angry, and I get even more angry when I think that the CEOs of these big chains of health clinics are getting bonuses of $10 million or $20 million because they managed to maximize profits—yet they managed to maximize profits by closing clinics to create an artificial scarcity, which now allows them to charge high prices for bad food and minimal therapy.

I left the clinic and drove to my mom's house and the whole way I kept thinking about how the slow consolidation of the health care clinics has been a disaster for U.S. health care. I recall when I was young, a number of political leaders insisted that if we privatize health care then we would end up with lower costs and higher quality because the health chains would be forced to compete. No one ever explained what would keep the private firms from closing enough clinics to create enough scarcity so they would be safe from competition, but of course, that's exactly what the major health chains did, because it's the obvious way to boost profits. Close clinics, create scarcity, raise prices.

P.S. I was about to send this and my mom called. She says she is miserable and she wants to go home tomorrow.

Subject: *we are told conflicting advice about health insurance*

Date: *January 14th, 2019*

Dear Kristin,

After I sent the previous email, my mom went to talk to the nurse. My mom told the nurse that she was going to leave tomorrow. The nurse said that if my mom left tomorrow then insurance wouldn't pay for any of the visit, so my mom would end up paying thousands of dollars. Therefore, my mom feels like she's stuck at this place, with the bad food and bad service and bad therapy. It seems like a scam.

I'm going there early tomorrow. At the very least, I will demand that my mom get more time in physical therapy, since that is the whole point of this. And I'll see if there is a way to get her out of there, assuming she still wants to go.

Subject: *everyone in my family has conflicting ideas about the next step, and it's chaos*

Date: *January 15, 2019*

Dear Natalie,

My brother Leonard called Mom. He seemed angry at the idea of her going home. He suggested she needed the physical therapy to get better. My brother Lance apparently feels the same. So my mom changed her mind and decided to stay. But I think that my brothers don't realize how miserable my mom is. We have to take care of her body, but also her spirit. If she's miserable, she won't get well. Now that she's taking oral antibiotics, she could take those at home just as well as at the clinic.

I'm going there today. And I'm bringing my mom some good food. If she has to stay there, I hope to make her feel comfortable.

Some thoughts written a year later
(This is no longer email.)

In total, my mom spent 6 weeks at the rehabilitation clinic. During that time, I believe she grew weaker, given that she was confined to her room for most of the day. She only got one exercise session per day, and during that session the physical therapist was often busy with other patients, so my mom ended up receiving only about 15 minutes of exercise a day. Though we'd been told the clinic would offer specialized training tailored to my mom, nothing of the sort ever happened. I regard the whole thing as a scam. Only towards the end, after I had complained to management, did the situation improve.

In January of 2019, it seemed unlikely that my mom had much more time to live. Even high doses of antibiotics were barely able to bring her pneumonia under control, and she was left with damaged lungs. I recall praying for her to live for one more year. I asked the heavens that we might be granted one more fun summer, one more trip to Charlottesville, one more visit with Misty and Kristin. I think on some level I was asking for some time to say goodbye. I was granted my wish.

My mom took another course of antibiotics that January, then and another in March, and then again in June and August. It seemed inevitable that the pneumonia would kill her. But then her doctor suggested she take vitamin D. This was a miracle. She hasn't been sick since she started taking vitamin D.

Apparently seniors suffer vitamin deficiencies that are much more severe than younger people. My friend Joanna Salidis, who studied neurology, told me of an old woman who was brought to her clinic. The woman's family had said that she had come down with dementia. The sudden onset was suspicious. First they ruled out a stroke. Then Joanna gave the woman some vitamin B. And voilà! The woman made a rapid recovery. This is a known problem: vitamin B deficiency leading to dementia in older people.

For my mom, her illness was resolved with vitamin D.

Anyway, I spent all of that year thinking that I was dealing with a short-term crisis. It is amazing that my mom recovered and is still alive, 17 months after those terrible days in the hospital.

Regarding my mom's illness, there were five main lessons that I'd like to summarize:

1. The squeaky wheel gets the oil.

I started to complain about the lack of attention that my mom was getting at the rehab clinic. The more I complained, the more they gave her attention. It's important to push these systems.

2. Worthless treatments.

Despite my best efforts, my mom never got more than 45

minutes of exercise a day at the rehab clinic. She was forced to spend most her time in bed. Every day that she was left to rot in that establishment left her weaker. Such clinics must have to check a box in the vast apparatus of the system that attempts to measure what health care is being delivered to each individual. If you were to design a system that starts with the essential health care principles, you would never create these rehabilitation clinics.

For most families and individuals, there is likely an alternative that is both cheaper and better, which is, let's figure out some exercise that the patient can do with a family member or friend or home health care professional, then offer some basic training, then release the patient into the care of that family member or ally. And for sure, the most important exercise that my mom needed was simply going for walks. Once she was released, we did a lot of walking. My mom and I walked several times a day.

At first, she could barely walk 100 meters, and I'd hold her hand to steady her. But after 2 weeks, she was able to walk 500 meters. After a month, she could walk a kilometer. By August of 2019, she was able to walk 2 kilometers and she no longer needed to lean on me. It was remarkable to see her regain her strength, despite her advanced age.

3. Fraud.

"If your mom leaves the rehabilitation clinic before she

is supposed to, the insurance company won't pay and you'll face a bill of many thousands of dollars." For the most part, this is a lie and a scam. I eventually did some research about this. Almost the opposite is true. It turns out that Medicare is wary of facilities that try to scam money from patients without offering much real physical therapy. You can call and report claims like my mother and I heard, and Medicare has a related unit that can investigate of such cases. While it is possible that Medicare will refuse to pay the rehabilitation clinic in cases of suspected fraud, my mom would never be exposed to any liability. The fight over payment would be entirely between Medicare and the clinic.

4. The children start fighting.

This was maybe the biggest surprise—the thing that I least expected. But perhaps it makes sense. When my father was nearing his end, my mom was there to make decisions for him, so I never ended up arguing with my brothers over the right strategy for my dad. But when my mom was at risk of dying, suddenly one of my brothers was full of opinions. He was too busy with work to come visit, but he called from San Francisco fairly often. He never had enough information to really understand the situation here on the East Coast, but, presumably out of fear and concern, he was trying to micromanage the situation from a distance. I felt strongly that all decisions had to be made by those of us who were there in the room, talking to the various medical professionals. That meant me and my mom, sometimes aided by my mom's minister. I give this advice to everyone: When you only have one parent left, make sure you know who will be making decisions in an emergency.

5. Power of attorney.

Make sure your parents have their paperwork up to date (and keep your own paperwork up to date). My mom and dad drew up their will and power of attorney documents when they were both healthy. My mom never updated them after my dad died. As such, decision-making became a shouting match among my siblings. Make sure everyone in your family updates their important paperwork after each major life event, such as a birth or a death. Among the other benefits, there should be clarity of responsibilities should a parent become incapacitated.

Eventually, I decided that my mom should move in with me. We sold the house in Jackson at the end of 2019. We traveled for a bit, and then settled into my apartment in New York City. We were, in fact, just settling in when Covid-19 bloomed into a global pandemic, and for a while New York City became the epicenter of the disease.

When your parents reach the end of their lives, your family will probably find itself in need of a person who is, in part, a lawyer, but also a nurse, a general practitioner, a family therapist, a medical ethicist, a spiritual leader, and a government bureaucrat with deep knowledge of all applicable government programs. What is the chance that you can find such a miracle worker? Sadly, such people don't really exist, but we are reaching a moment when we'll all need such a specialty to be invented. Until then, I must recommend that each of you try to develop relationships with professionals who might be able to fill in at least some of the gaps.

Part III

A Possible Reform

After all the troubles my family has had with the modern medical bureaucracy, I've come to believe it is essential that every person have a patient-advocate for their journey through such a system.

First let me back up a little and explain why I think the current system is failing people. The growing complexity of modern technologies and the increasing specialization occurring within the medical field have wrought changes in the bureaucracy, which in turn have wrought changes in the way ordinary people interact with medical professionals. In some ways, unfortunately, our cultural assumptions about medical care remain stuck in a previous century. In particular, we assume that the goodwill of ordinary doctors and nurses is enough to overcome the inertia which is a natural part of all bureaucracies. Changing circumstances increasingly means that this assumption is deadly.

What's the difference between a patient-advocate and a doctor? Most people go into the medical field at least in part because they want to help others, so it seems reasonable to assume goodwill on the part of everyone in medicine. It therefore seems unreasonable to introduce an element into the doctor-patient relationship which might be seen as adversarial. But let's examine this. Would a patient-advocate necessarily have to be adversarial toward doctors? Even if the answer were "yes," is it always a bad thing to set up a relationship with the potential for conflict?

Consider the law, courts, or politics. Allowing defendants to hire lawyers to represent them in court is now universally recognized as a human right. And most of us feel that democratic debate is made more inclusive when multiple voices are free to battle it out and advance different narratives. So theoretically, a diversity of opinions ensures that the best ideas are brought forward.

While this concept may be controversial, I believe it's important to encourage a similar model for medical care.

I have many friends who are doctors or nurses, and I know how they would respond. "We go to work every day hoping to help people, and our only concern is achieving the best possible outcomes for our patients."

I'm sure that that is true. For a long time, I was close to a woman who was a nurse, and she was utterly dedicated to her patients. She fought for each of them. She cried whenever someone passed away. No reasonable person can doubt that most medical professionals are genuine crusaders for the good health of those they serve.

Yet in the 21st century, we have a wealth of psychological studies that reveal how much an individual's effort can be distorted by group dynamics. (Consider the original Milgram experiments in the 1960s where participants believed they were delivering possibly lethal electric shocks to study subjects, and these participants did so feeling that those in charge of the study would accept responsibility for such cruelty. Workers in bureaucracies often demonstrate this same obedience to rules, even when their actions lead to unfortunate results. See *https://www.verywellmind.com/the-milgram-obedience-experiment-2795243*.) Every system develops its own dynamics, which often limit the effectiveness of the people being managed. Occasionally, these dynamics result in outcomes utterly unlike what people in the system actually want. Therefore, accepting and encouraging professional differences of opinion will probably lead to better results for patients.

This principle is already recognized regarding pregnancy, where it's common for women to have a doula in the birthing room — someone who is trained to advocate for them. I'm suggesting that something similar needs to be expanded to all patients, in all situations. Consider my own story, as I interacted with the medical establishment to advocate for my father and later my mother: I did not *want* to be adversarial, but occasionally I had to be, in order to get the best care for my parents. Unfortunately I lacked the training to be as effective as I could have been, which is why I now believe we must have professional patient-advocates.

Accepting patient-advocates as a normal part of all medical care would offer two benefits:

1. Education. Patients who know nothing about the med-

ical system would have an objective professional who could explain the system to them. This professional would not be captive to any particular branch of medicine. This approach also holds the potential to avoid wasted effort and therefore save healthcare costs.

2. Advocacy. When a blind algorithm, enforced by an unthinking bureaucracy, would lead to a horrific outcome for a particular patient, there would be someone with a deep understanding of the processes of that bureaucracy who could stand up against it.

Am I actually suggesting something new? One could argue that anyone in the U.S. can hire a lawyer and sue any medical establishment for malpractice. In this sense, what I'm suggesting already exists. But malpractice lawsuits are reactive; they happen *after* something problematic has taken place. I'm proposing something much more proactive — a process that helps shape the care a patient receives while they're in the hospital or receiving treatment on an outpatient basis.

What's the difference between a patient-advocate and a doctor? During the 1800s, a doctor was someone who took absolute responsibility for the health of a family. At that time, a family doctor was practically part of the family. If someone was sick, you called the doctor and they came over to your house to see if they could help.

We have been moved away from that model by two related factors:

1. The growth of medical knowledge has, since then, led to specialization among medical professionals.

2. A vast bureaucracy sprang up to organize the different specialists and to manage the money needed to pay for the complexity of the services within the system.

Consider the novel *Tristram Shandy* written by Laurence Sterne and published in 1759. In the book, Sterne muses that doctors are making such remarkable discoveries, at such an astonishing speed, that the sum total of all medical knowledge actually doubled during the previous seven years. I'm not sure how he was measuring, but it is true that things were moving quickly at that time and have continued to do so for the ensuing 262 years.

By 1900, it was generally understood that the total amount of medical knowledge was exceeding what one person could memorize, even if they devoted their whole life to study; therefore, doctors were going to have to specialize. And as they specialized, they began to lose sight of patients as whole people and instead came to see them as blobs of specialty parts: a heart, a liver, a nervous system. The most obvious evidence for this is how quickly doctors now refer you to another specialist, as soon as they believe your problem is not covered by their specialty. I do not mean to make this sound like a personal failing; rather, this is simply how specialization works, in all fields. An estate lawyer can write you a will, but they won't have a conjecture of the outcome if you happen to be on trial for murder. A marriage counselor can guide a conversation between you and your spouse but won't typically feel qualified to help you with your drug addiction. The modern world is a world of specialists. We gain some benefits from this, but there are also a number of costs.

The crucial point is that we no longer have doctors as they were in the 1800s. Most people make the assumption that the modern general practitioner (GP) is the same as what used to simply be called "doctor," but there are some important distinctions. In particular, a GP typically won't offer guidance if you get contradictory advice from two different specialists.

Here's an example. You're a middle-age male with some occasional chest discomfort. You go see your GP, who sends you to a cardiologist. The cardiologist says your arteries are clogged and you'll have to go for triple bypass surgery. You're concerned and you'd like to know your options. Both your GP and the cardiologist suggest you get a second opinion. So you go and see a second cardiologist. This new cardiologist doesn't think your condition is so bad and suggests that it can be managed with medication; no surgery is necessary.

Who is right? And who can help you decide? If you ask the GP, they demur and explain that they cannot advise against a cardiologist on a matter explicitly involving the heart.

You can seek a third opinion, a fourth, a fifth. You'll end

up with a lot of opinions. And in the end the decision will be yours to make.

That's what I find amazing regarding the modern medical system. On the most complex issues of life and death, we are made to rely on our own resources.

I'd like to share another example. At the end of 2019, my mom and I decided that we should sell her house and that she should move in with me. We assumed that my mom would spend some of each month with me, and alternately some time at a retirement home. But then the coronavirus pandemic swept across the globe and elder care facilities became hotspots, so that was no longer an option. Nor did I have the ability to take care of her full-time. A friend in Virginia who used to be a nurse suggested we head south and live with her for a while. This was when New York had been badly hit, and Virginia seemed untouched.

A month later, however, the number of cases in New York was rapidly declining, whereas in Virginia it was rising. New questions to consider arose. How bad might the epidemic get in Virginia? If we went there, did that mean Mom was giving up on regular physical therapy? If we stayed a long time, would Mom have to find new doctors?

A few other options seemed worth exploring. What if Mom went to live with her best friend Laurie for a while? The two had met at Hunter College in 1946 and were still friends even now, and Laurie was still healthy and drove her own car. She had a spacious house in New Jersey. But what if there were some kind of calamity? What if Mom fell again? Would that be too large a responsibility to put on her elderly friend?

In this scenario, there were many benefits and risks to consider. How should we decide? Few GPs would feel comfortable commenting on such nuanced issues. In a world of medical specialists, families have to make the most important decisions without any help from medical professionals. While a family might have a very good relationship with a particular doctor, who might have opinions on these complex questions, many doctors would be cautious about giving a professional opinion on a set of questions which partly concern matters that are not strictly medical.

What is needed is someone neutral — someone a bit outside the medical system, but who understands it well.

The role of patient-advocate would combine attributes of a doula, a lawyer, and some old functions of a family doctor.

There is one more trend to consider which influenced how I reached my conclusions.

Around 1900, doctors spent close to 0% of their time on paperwork. They might quickly dictate some notes to a nurse, who would act as secretary. There was no bureaucracy and no managing payment systems, so there was no need to figure out which "codes" the bureaucracy was expecting for a given condition, treatment, or test.

In the 1960s, American doctors were still only spending about 5% of their time on paperwork, though with the growth of private insurance and the introduction of Medicare and then Medicaid, the need for paperwork was growing. Fortunately most insurance schemes at this time covered 100% of costs without review, so there was no system of approval needed, no co-pays, no complex math regarding who had to cover what percentage of each different procedure.

In the early 1990s, health maintenance organizations (HMOs) began to take over, and with it the concept of "managed care," which was a euphemism for insurance companies that could argue over a bill and refuse payment for some procedures. This meant doctors now had to justify, document — and in some cases, ask permission for enacting — the care they deemed best for their patients. This was the inflection point that led to the explosion of bureaucracy. Even worse, most small hospitals didn't have the money to hire lawyers to fight the HMOs when they refused payment. The biggest medical systems, however, did have the money to hire such lawyers and win cases ... awarding them even more money. It was the beginning of the era when the American medical system began to consolidate. Small, rural hospitals no longer generated enough revenue to survive.

Currently, studies suggest doctors are spending almost 50% of their time on paperwork. When economists wonder, "Why has labor productivity in the U.S. stagnated for the last 50 years?" they should consider situations like this, in which the best-educated and most productive category of worker loses 50% of their time to paperwork. Among the many problems of the complex payment situation, it has amounted to a war against efficiency.

In recent years, the system has been relying more frequently on nurse practitioners (NPs) instead of doctors. For instance, a nurse practitioner anesthesiologist does everything that an anesthesiologist used to do — but the anesthesiologist continues to carry the legal burden and the insurance to protect them from lawsuits, while the NP does all of the work. During surgery, a nurse practitioner anesthesiologist will keep the patient alive. In theory, the NP is under the authority of the actual anesthesiologist, but this is mostly a legal fiction (outside of a crisis).

While this system can be applauded for separating the medical work from the legal burdens of the work, it means that a doctor spends 10 to 15 years learning a specialty, such as anesthesiology, and then immediately abandons it and becomes a manager who oversees nurse practitioners. Does that make sense? Can 15 years of study be justified if the goal is simply to satisfy some legal fiction? This seems unsustainable. For this reason, I view the current situation as transitional. But that raises the question, to what kind of system are we transitioning?

Start with the history, and then follow the trend. At some point, it's plausible that doctors will spend 70% of their time on paperwork, then 80%, then 90%, then eventually all of their time. The system is clearly demanding someone who can fill this role — someone who can absorb the legal burdens of the bureaucracy.

What does this mean? Why should the system generate such a curious and counterintuitive phenomenon? Why would anyone want doctors to spend almost all of their time on paperwork? At what point does the medical system actually return its focus to helping real human beings?

When I talk this over with friends who understand the medical system, some indulge in fantasy, believing that one day the bureaucracy will magically disappear. They suggest that in the future, the U.S. will have different payment mechanisms, perhaps single-payer, or perhaps whatever Sweden does, or Canada, and all of our problems will be solved once we pass a particular law.

While we can expect some progress towards universal payment of healthcare, reducing the bureaucracy is a fantasy. It is true that if the U.S. adopts a simple payment mechanism, then the bureaucracy will shrink, insofar as it relates to billing and payments. But it will continue to grow insofar as it relates to organizing an increasingly specialized system.

There are some counter arguments to consider. What if Artificial Intelligence (AI) and advanced robotics takes on more of the work that doctors do? Won't that reverse the trend? Since I am a software developer and I've worked on some AI projects, I believe I have some understanding of how these are usually applied. While robotics and AI can reduce some of the manual work, they rely on teams of computer programmers and data analysts to improve the statistical models on which they rely. In other words, rather than simplifying the system, they introduce more complexity. There might come a day, perhaps 50 years from now, when robot surgeons are a mature and stable technology, and at that time they might help simplify hospital work — but for now such speculation is pure science fiction. These new technologies are immature and undergoing rapid evolution, and as such, they demand large teams to maintain and update them. Therefore, they currently increase the burdens on the bureaucracy, and they increase the amount of specialization occurring in the overall system.

Therefore I take two trends to be irreversible:

1. Medical knowledge will continue to expand; ergo, medical professionals will continue to specialize into ever-narrower domains of knowledge.

2. The bureaucracy must continue to expand to help organize the complexity of a system that is made up of a number of increasingly narrow specialties.

I am somewhat influenced here by my long career in software development. A simple app can do one thing, do it well, and can be written in a day — and it can do a beautiful job with its one task. However, as a software system becomes more complex, a greater percentage of the system needs to be given over to the meta task of managing the system. In very large systems, one needs a system of systems. And as some of the systems I've worked on have been in the service of medical bureaucracies, the growth of the complexity of the software system has offered me insight into the growth of the complexity of such bureaucracies.

Is there any point having a doctor who spends 100% of their time on paperwork? Does it make sense that someone should spend 10 or 15 years of their life pursuing advanced medical skills, only to then be told that they should never again examine a human being? Doctors are, in some sense, the last guild of craftspeople. Even as advancing technology, increasing specialization, and mass production have virtually eliminated many of the great crafts of old — woodworking, glass-blowing, weaving — the same factors are eliminating the traditional role of general practitioners.

(I worry I will be misunderstood here: there is now a thing called "general practitioner," and perhaps there will always be a job role with that title. However, I'm saying that the role has narrowed so much that what "general practitioner" means now is different from what it used to mean; the job as it existed 100 years ago has been eliminated.)

It's possible that, just as the last craftspeople have largely disappeared from our economy, the doctor-as-craftsperson will also cease to exist. In the future, there will be patient-advocates and there will be medical specialists, the equivalent of nurse practitioners. Nothing else.

Often when I propose this possibility, the following exchange unfolds: In response to my idea someone will say, "Surely a person should rely on their doctor to make medical decisions!" Then, when I ask, "But what should happen when two doctors disagree?" they stumble, as if they haven't considered this circumstance, despite the fact that it's quite common in a society where having a second opinion on serious matters is the norm.

For any proposed change in the system, questions about the cost are valid. Would patient-advocates increase costs or would the gain in efficiency pay for itself? This deserves further study. What we can say right now, with certainty, is that the loss of doctors productivity is one of the things driving up costs, so anything that can take the burden of the bureaucracy away from doctors is a reform that deserves attention.

How should people get a diagnosis for their symptoms?

The American medical system works reasonably well when a person can easily be diagnosed and sent to a specialist in that particular disease or disorder. For example, a patient has an uneven, black skin lesion their GP recognizes as a potential melanoma. The GP sends them to an oncologist for further evaluation.

The American medical system does poorly when only a specialist would be able to make a diagnosis. Missing is the kind of meta system which might possess the knowledge to know which kind of knowledge is needed. I recently had a friend who initially thought she was having a heart attack, but later the doctors found elevated liver enzymes and what they thought was pneumonia. Then later they decided it might have been some kind of edema downstream of a cardiac event. In addition, her TSH levels were off so they decided she was hypothyroid. Later still, it was decided the real cause of all the symptoms was perhaps an adrenal crisis leading to a lack of cortisol, which set off a whole cascade of other events. Over the course of six weeks, she went to the emergency room ten times and visited numerous specialists, all of whom gave her a different diagnosis. In the end she primarily had to figure the problem out herself, and she realized that she needed to see an endocrinologist.

After a long series of emails in which she described her situation to me, I wrote to her:

"The medical system nearly lost you in its maze of narrow specialists. There was some doctor, somewhere in the system, who could have given you the correct diagnosis, but the system itself did not know how to connect you with that doctor. This was a failure of the meta system, the system that oversees the higher-level functions of the medical system. It failed you because it barely exists, and it barely exists because we rarely talk about how important it has become in a world full of narrow specialists. Because if the system is ignorant of what you need, as a practical matter, the result is the same as if every doctor were ignorant of what you need. Without a better guidance system to connect patients to the correct specialist, the patients will never get a correct diagnosis.

And yet our medical system proceeds on the basis that everything should go in the opposite direction: first you should get a correct diagnosis and then you will be sent to the correct specialist."

Another, related problem is when a patient has several symptoms, but a doctor becomes fixated on a single one of those symptoms. The friend, who I just mentioned, took a list of nine symptoms to her doctor. The first symptom was a sudden neck pain. The doctor fixated on that. Ignoring the other symptoms (elevated liver enzymes, a racing heart, pneumonia), the doctor became convinced that my friend had a pinched nerve in her neck. A rationalist might warn us of "confirmation bias," the mistake of locking on to a pattern too quickly. Perhaps the doctor had recently seen another patient who had a pinched nerve, so now the doctor thought everyone had a pinched nerve. It's a well-known cognitive bias.

One thing that might fix this situation is having a team of people who diagnose patients. A team of three or more would allow each person to balance the quirks and specialties of the others on the team. In theory, this should lead to a balanced assessment of what a patient is actually struggling with. Having specialists who only focus on the task of diagnosis might help fix the problem of our failing meta system, that is, the outer system that should tell a patient which kind of specialist they need to go see in the inner system. But it seems expensive and unlikely that one could get three or more doctors together in a room to diagnose someone. An implication is that these two changes are related and need to be implemented simultaneously:

1. Diagnosis needs to become a specialty, with teams of less trained, less expensive diagnosticians working together to achieve better results than what could be achieved by a single doctor, even if that single doctor was a superstar of unusual talent.

2. Having at least three diagnosticians would help balance the process of reaching a conclusion. Even if one of them latches onto a symptom and begins to speak tangentially, the other two could push back and bring up alternative possibilities.

But just as doctors disagree, three diagnosticians will inevitably also have disagreements. So again the question would surface, how should a decision be made when a patient is faced with multiple medical opinions?

The patient-advocate is the modern day doctor.

Coming full circle, I'm left with the conclusion that a patient-advocate should be what in the 1800s was called a "doctor." That is, someone who takes absolute responsibility for the health of an individual and their family — someone who is practically a part of the family. Unlike doctors of old, a patient-advocate wouldn't perform any medical procedures; rather, just as a good lawyer knows how to navigate the courts, the patient-advocate would know how to navigate the medical bureaucracy so as to bring forth the resources you need.

Perhaps you need a cardiologist, or a fertility specialist, or a CAT scan. Perhaps you need a knowledgeable professional to represent your interests to an endocrinologist regarding the possibility that you're one of the many people who suffer a non-standard presentation of hypothyroidism. When your cardiologist, in turn, says you need surgery, you'll want a second and third opinion — and you may be given conflicting advice. There's a joke that if you assemble ten doctors in a room and ask them about a medical problem you'll get twelve opinions. Your patient-advocate is the objective voice you turn to for help when making difficult decisions about whose opinion you can most trust.

What is the appropriate education for a patient-advocate? The patient-advocate must have a medical education, but not necessarily one as lengthy as that of a doctor. They should have an extensive understanding of medicine, but also the organizational skills of an executive assistant, a personal chief-of-staff, and occasionally the argumentative skills of a good lawyer. The education of an ideal patient-advocate would cover some of the same things doctors learn, such as medical ethics, but it would require a more extensive study. Finally, the perfect patient-advocate is one who studies decision-making under stress, as that is exactly what most families face when they face the medical system — and rarely have they had the proper training to handle the difficulties of such decisions.

Once such a patient-advocate role is established as a norm of the medical system (as commonplace as a person hiring a lawyer when they must go to court), then some of the relationship that once existed between doctors and patients can become a relationship between doctors and patient-advocates, and then the relationship between a patient-advocate and patient can absorb some of the dynamics which had once been more directly between patient and doctor. A family would then receive medical news from someone with a long-standing relationship with them, someone who knows how to talk to them. I mean this both literally, as in a family who speaks Spanish or Hindi would have a patient-advocate who speaks Spanish or Hindi, but also figuratively. When my mom fell and hurt herself, we went to one hospital, then another, then a rehabilitation clinic, and during those weeks I spoke to at least nine doctors. It seemed like every day we were talking to someone entirely new, someone who was learning my mom's history for the first time. Having a patient-advocate of long standing between us and the doctors would have been an immense relief.

(This essay would be much longer if I tried to tackle the question of gender, as well as the enormous amount of sexism in the system. One thing that made my family's experience somewhat unique is that my parents only had sons.

No daughters. And over and over again I was struck by the way that the medical system assumes that every family has a young-ish healthy person who is not working, someone with a flexible schedule who can take an ailing parent to an appointment at any time of the day. This assumption might have worked in the 1950s but it does not work now. The assumption that there is a wife or daughter or daughter-in-law who is not working is simply unsustainable in the modern world. Thus another argument for patient-advocates is that they would professionalize the many tasks that the medical system anachronistically assumes it can leave to the women in the family.)

Furthermore, much of the burden of paperwork can be moved from the doctors to the patient-advocates. Perhaps patient-advocates can be legally authorized to write up summaries of the information that they hear from the various doctors. After all, someone in the system should take legal responsibility for the medical advice a patient hears, even when different doctors are giving conflicting advice.

When I share these ideas with friends, some of them suggest that I'm describing a dark dystopia in which patients and doctors view each other as enemies. Wouldn't it be better, they ask, to live in a world where the family doctor gets to know everyone in the family? Surely we want our doctor to also be our friend? That sounds correct, and where possible, we should want a trusting relationship with those who help us with life-and-death situations. But let's think carefully about what is possible, in general, for the average person in the overall system.

We have gained some things from the increasing specialization of medicine. 150 years ago, doctors could not treat cancer; later, after World War I, a family could go to a general family doctor who knew something about the first chemotherapy treatments. As science led to additional breakthroughs, seeing a radiologist or a chemotherapist, each with their specialties, became possible. And more recently, a woman with breast cancer might have the option to see a breast cancer specialist who would know, for instance, the appropriate timing to try prescribing Tamoxifen. Every step toward specialization has increased the possible efficacy of the treatment. How many of us would be willing to give that up to go back to some nostalgic paradise where our doctors got to know us as good personal friends?

Anyone who watches television is aware how strongly Americans dream of perfect doctors. Perhaps it's Alan Alda's charismatic and empathetic Hawkeye Pierce on *M*A*S*H* back in the 1970s; George Clooney's character in *ER* in the 1990s; Jane Seymour as *Medicine Woman*, also in the 1990s; Hugh Laurie as Dr. Gregory House in the 2000s; or the cast of the never-ending *Grey's Anatomy*. Regardless, it's clear that medical miracles are among the country's most fervent of fantasies. This is completely understandable: none of us wants to die.

In a medical crisis, we all want to believe that there is a

doctor out there, somewhere, who can take one look at us and immediately identify the problem and the cure. However, when we think of the kind of system we want in the real world, it's important to set our fantasies aside. Superstars are difficult to find, but even if they were common, teams of closely coordinated specialists tend to beat singular superstars. If we can free our minds from nostalgia and look plainly at the trends of the last 50 years, it's clear that the only way to take advantage of the growth of medical knowledge is by finding better ways to integrate the skills of many narrowly focused practitioners.

It will be critically important that we achieve the "closely coordinated" aspect of the new model. It's not a job that can be handled by a GP, since the task of closely coordinating medical specialists needs to be handled by someone who can come along with the patient when they are meeting with various medical professionals.

As said before, our medical system optimizes for certain straightforward situations. If you are a middle-age man with chest pain, you're lucky to be in the U.S. If you are a middle-age woman with vague neurological pains, you may be out of luck. Over the course of two years, you may be sent to a dozen different specialists, each of whom might have a different diagnosis for you. One might tell you that you have hypothyroidism, another may suggest that it's Crohn's disease, and a third may say it is fibromyalgia or Lyme disease. Ask ten doctors and you'll get twelve opinions, but you won't be offered a disciplined, structured process for narrowing those twelve opinions down to one or two action items that deserve to be prioritized over the others. But assuming that the medical profession eventually develops a disciplined, structured process for prioritizing those action items — who will explain it to you, who will walk you through the process, and who will organize all of the actual follow-up work?

People who've never had a complex illness don't realize what a nightmare the American medical system can be, not just because of the complicated insurance situation, but also because it's so common for one doctor to send you to another doctor, who in turn sends you to another doctor. And in the event each of them has the next six weeks booked solid, you may find yourself waiting a month or two for an appointment ... then another month for another appointment with someone else ... and a year goes by and you've made only minor progress toward getting a real answer to your questions. And meanwhile you feel worse and worse.

What will the American medical system look like in 50 years? Has the national leadership done a good job of leading the nation in a conversation about how the system will change?

Anyone who has read much economic history knows that a team of narrowly focused specialists can often deliver a faster, higher-quality, lower-cost product than what is delivered by a master craftsperson. Adam Smith gave us the example of a pin factory where every worker did a single thing (one draws the metal out, another sharpens the point, another applies the head, and so forth). Each worker therefore performed that one job better and faster than they could have possibly done if they were trying to make an entire pin, so the pin factory produced many more pins as a result. A century later, Henry Ford offered another example of essentially the same phenomenon by producing cars on an assembly line, with each worker performing a specific task. Suddenly, cars were cheaper and better quality than the cars that were built slowly by master craftspeople. Surely something similar must eventually happen in the medical care system. The level of specialization continues to increase, but so far the work is still mandated, by legal edict, to follow a process that first took shape in the late 1800s, with a single doctor carrying nominal legal authority to authorize each step in the process. How long can that old system continue to work? Do we want it to continue? Will we be happy if the same process is still in place 50 years from now?

Sadly, in the U.S., the financial question uses up everyone's energy. We've wasted decades arguing over who will pay for healthcare. I am hopeful that at some point the progressives will win on this issue, simply because it would allow us to talk about the other important aspects of the medical system. If we end up with universal health care (be it single-payer, Medicaid For All, Medicare For All, or subsidized insurance) then we can confront the next great question, which pertains to what sort of changes we would like to see in the relationship between medical professionals and patients.

I am not suggesting that introducing patient-advocates into the system, as a regular and accepted feature of the system, would lead us to utopia. I'm only saying it is, at this point, a necessary reform, because ordinary people cannot easily understand how to navigate the complexity of the system, and increasing specialization among doctors means that doctors are no longer able to play their old role. Nor would it be correct to say, "Your GP is supposed to play the role that you are describing." That is not even close to being correct. What is needed is someone who will sit with the patient, in the hospital room, and talk over all of the information that the doctors have just delivered.

Clearly, the system has evolved to such a point that it demands a general re-write of the relationships between actors in the medical system. An expansive patient-advocate role could unburden doctors and lead to an improvement in the productivity of the system, while at the same time giving families the crucial perspective needed to make difficult decisions.

...

In this book I have described two crucial moments in my family's medical history, one of which I got wrong and one of which I got right:

Wrong — thinking that my father might survive for a few more months or years, when in fact he had a week left.

Right — forgoing a possibly fatal surgery which had no hope of restoring my mother's eyesight.

In the latter situation, I played the role of patient-advocate ... but I did so without training, uncertain and afraid, forced to fight a system without the experience or information that could have offered a much greater degree of confidence that I was making the right decision.

It is not utopian to think that a patient-advocate would have told us the truth in the first situation and would have made the second much easier. And I believe a patient-advocate can help you and your family, just as much as a patient-advocate could have helped mine.

You might well be wiser than I am, dear reader. At least, I hope so. But remember that when you are facing the suffering of a loved one, you may not be thinking clearly. And in such situations, you might be grateful for someone who can do your thinking for you, and fight for you, and fight for your family, and defend your loved ones till the last moment that our mortal efforts might be able to help them.

To learn more about the career of the photographer Ralph Krubner, check out the following article, "Ramblin Ralph," from the August, 1984 edition of the magazine *American Photographer.*

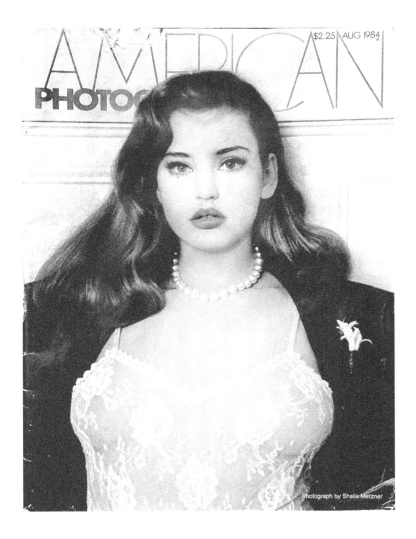

Ramblin' Ralph

Searching for the ordinary image is the extraordinary way Ralph Krubner makes a living.
by Terri Jentz

The walls of Ralph Krubner's house in Jackson, New Jersey are lined with cardboard picture puzzles framed in gold. The puzzles have earned their place of honor, not because the Krubner children succeeded in putting them together, but because Ralph Krubner shot the photographs from which the puzzles are made. These charming vistas include: the quaintest possible fishing village in Nova Scotia, a brick-red sawmill complete with waterfall, and a snow-capped peak offset by a perfectly gnarled and weathered tree.

All of Krubner's images are what you might call picture perfect. He is one of a handful of professional photographers who shoots almost exclusively for stock, creating all-purpose pictures that are designed to fit an optimum number of uses. They appear in every conceivable format—from calendars to seed catalogs to sticky greeting cards. Unlike editorial and advertising photographers who shoot to fill specific needs of editors and art directors, Krubner must create his own assignments. His job is to anticipate which images, colors and compositions will have the most applications, and then produce them. Krubner's carefully crafted images then go on file at H. Armstrong Roberts, a stock agency based in Philadelphia. In exchange for a percentage, the agency sells the shots to a wide variety of clients who put them on everything from catalogues to travel posters.

The qualifier "stock" before the word photography has a distinctly unglamourous ring when compared to such chic pursuits as art, advertising and

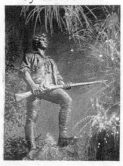

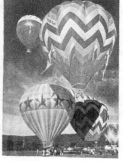

fashion. But unglamourous does not necessarily equal unprofitable. It is difficult to ascertain how much money is made annually on stock photography in this country, as most stock agencies are closely held corporations which are competitive and highly secretive about their sales figures. Industry experts estimate that stock sales may well gross $20,000,000 a year, if one considers the many branches of stock photography. These include agencies like Roberts which sells to low-end editorial and commercial clients; the giant stock houses like Image Bank, 4 × 5 and Photofile International offering more exotic images to high-paying advertising agencies, and the editorial stock houses like Woodfin Camp Associates and Photo Researchers whose major markets are slick magazines and high-quality books.

Many big-name photographers derive considerable income either from private sales of their stock, or through stock houses. Pete Turner and Jay Maisel, for example, learned long ago that

(At top) The Minuteman statue in Lexington, Massachusetts, was shot with a 4 × 5 in 1976, during the bicentennial celebration. Krubner added the fireworks in the darkroom using the bursts from several different chromes. (At left) The balloons have been used to illustrate a variety of concepts. They appear on "Have a Happy Day" greeting cards as well as in many ads. (Opposite) Ralph Krubner poses with a favorite skyline.

48

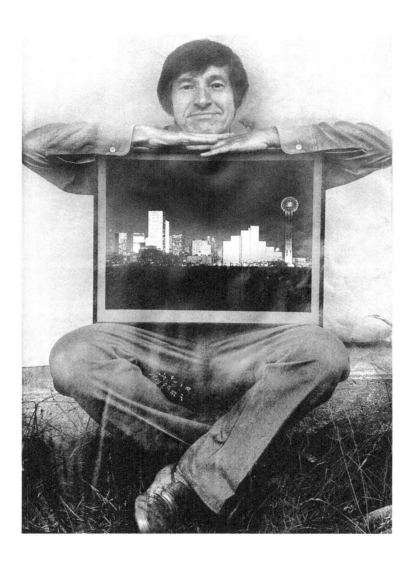

Text below has been transcribed from original.

Ramblin' Ralph

*Searching for the ordinary image is
the extraordinary way Ralph Krubner makes a living.*
By Terri Jentz
American Photographer, August 1984.

The walls of Ralph Krubner's house in Jackson, New Jersey are
lined with cardboard picture puzzles framed in gold. The puzzles
have earned their place of honor, not because the Krubner children
succeeded in putting them together, but because Ralph Krubner shot
the photographs from which the puzzles are made. These charming
vistas include: the quaintest possible fishing village in Nova Scotia, a
brick-red sawmill complete with waterfall, and a snow-capped peak
offset by a perfectly gnarled and weathered tree.

All of Krubner's images are what you might call picture perfect.
He is one of a handful of professional photographers who shoots
almost exclusively for stock, creating all-purpose pictures that are
designed to fit an optimum number of uses. They appear in every
conceivable format - from calendars to seed catalogs to sticky greeting
cards. Unlike editorial and advertising photographers who shoot to
fill specific needs of editors and art directors, Krubner must create his
own assignments. His job is to anticipate which images, colors and
compositions will have the most applications, and then produce them.
Krubner's carefully crafted images then go on file at H. Armstrong
Roberts, a stock agency based in Philadelphia. In exchange for a
percentage, the agency sells the shots to a wide variety of clients who
put them on everything from catalogues to travel posters.

The qualifier "stock" before the word photography has a distinctly unglamourous ring when compared to such chic pursuits as
art, advertising and fashion. But unglamourous does not necessarily
equal unprofitable. It is difficult to ascertain how much money is
made annually on stock photography in this country, as most stock
agencies are closely held corporations which are competitive and
highly secretive about their sales figures. Industry experts estimate
that stock sales may well gross $20,000,000 a year, if one considers

the many branches of stock photography. These include agencies like
Roberts which sells to low-end editorial and commercial clients; the
giant stock houses like Image Bank, 4 x 5 and Photofile International
offering more exotic images to high-paying advertising agencies, and
the editorial stock houses like Woodfin Camp Associates and Photo
Researchers whose major markets are slick magazines and high-qual-
ity books.

Many big-name photographers derive considerable income
either from private sales of their stock, or through stock houses. Pete
Turner and Jay Maisel, for example, learned long ago that their out-
takes can be turned into a steady stream of cash, and their vacations
can become tax-deductible "stock shooting trips."

Turner has some 2,000 slides on file at the Image Bank.
Through its New York office and 24 foreign franchises, Image Bank
grosses half a million dollars on Turner's work alone. Of this, Turner
netted last year about $140,000 - what he calls "not a bad piece of
change" for a sidelight to his assignment work. But it is Turner's
assignment work that has won him his international reputation; for
the photographer who shoots only stock, recognition does not come
easily, if at all. While he is no Pete Turner, Krubner has a stock file
of 70,000 images and has been published - by his own estimate -
more than 14,800 times! Yet in a 25-year career he has had only
a few dozen credit lines. The purple first-place ribbons from the
Ocean County Camera Club that line his darkroom walls are the
only official recognition he has won. "The situation is a little annoy-
ing," Krubner admits.

Krubner's darkroom is stuffed with neatly labeled files that read
like products in the generic aisle of a supermarket: "crowds, holidays,
sports, entertainment, offices, schools…." Krubner aims to make
ideal or typical pictures. "I've always got to get a perfect lawn," he
explains. "If they're selling weed killer or grass seed, one dande-
lion and the picture is out." In fact, Krubner's best-selling image
was made on his own suburban lawn. It is a close-up of a monarch
butterfly perched on a flower. "It has been said that a good stock
photograph is just a cliché." Ralph philosophizes. "Then the best
we can hope for is to find the next new cliché." Krubner admits that
much of what he shoots is "really humdrum," but on the other hand,
his lifestyle and mode of working indicate that finding the humdrum
can be fun, as well as a challenge.

One of the joys of stock shooting is the freedom it allows. Krubner gets to work without an art director breathing down his neck, and has never been shouted at over the phone by an editor. If he feels like working near home, he can book models and set up a shoot, right in his own neighborhood, conveniently located near the Jersey shore. If the weather is right ("sunny and hazy is good for models - there are no harsh shadows and no squinty expressions"), he may shoot a model jogging along a footpath, or a couple hand-in-hand on the boardwalk. More complicated shoots involve props like the car and luggage he used for a recent "packing the car" illustration. If the weather's bad, there are always indoor locations, like a nearby health club which, like the shot of the runner, will help fill the current demand for health and fitness pictures.

Krubner is quick to point out that not all stock shots are made on perfect days. "A snowstorm is great for weather shots," he says, and also emphasizes the importance of the unexpected. For instance, on a recent trip to the Southwest, Krubner stopped outside Austin, Texas, where he saw some beautiful cloud formations. "I grabbed my 4 x 5 and just started shooting," says Krubner, "and those pictures sold more than everything else from the whole trip combined." Krubner is also accustomed to revisiting old locations in search of new material. He can shoot where he likes, when he likes, and in the spring Krubner likes to go to Philadelphia.

It's early May, and Ralph, who looks a little like Leonard Nimoy with his hair swept forward over elfish ears, is driving into Philadelphia from the north, through a thicket of oil refineries. En route to a city not generally praised for its scenic glories, Krubner is determined to make pretty transparencies destined for travel brochures. He pulls into the center of town where a fire had recently ravaged a four-block section of the city. The smoky wasteland, a perfect set for a new wave fashion shoot or a punk rock video, holds no appeal for Krubner. With his cameras swinging on embroidered straps, he gingerly hops over the police barricades and passes the rubble on his way to a more photogenic attraction: the decorative pagoda that welcomes tourists to Chinatown. Using the shadow of his head on the pavement, Krubner calculates the position of the sun to determine shadow detail and zooms in for a tight shot of gold and red dragons high above.

Elsewhere in the City of Brotherly Love, Krubner carefully avoids such imperfections as fat ladies in shorts and people in
wheelchairs. He favors typical people in crisp new spring clothes.
"Do I want that blonde in the tight jeans enough to put up with the
guy in the Bermuda shorts?" Krubner wonders aloud as he shoots a
renovated street in Society Hill complete with gaslights, cobblestones
and an "apothecary." Krubner doesn't know what he'll do with the
shots of the Rosicrucian street magician with a drugged rabbit. But
he "shoots him because he's there," to satisfy his photojournalistic
instinct. Krubner admits that his branch of photography is not the
most creative, and for the most part, his quirky, idiosyncratic shots
don't sell. "I wanted to be a photojournalist once," he laments,
"back in the days when no one had even heard of stock photography.
Everybody wanted to work for *Life*, but I just couldn't get in. After a
while I had to go with what worked. Was it John Lennon who said
"Life is what happens when you're waiting for what you dreamed
of…?" He trails off, unable to recall the lyric. "Anyway, you wind up
doing the possible."

Krubner's wife Blanche, a red-haired dynamo who teaches high
school history and also hosts her own local cable TV show, thinks that
Krubner could stand to be more inventive. "I happen to feel that
Ralph is a lot more creative than he allows himself to be. He concen-
trates too much on getting a return on his investment." But Blanche
admits that "considering my personality, I'm lucky that I married the
man I did." Blanche appreciates the luxury of a freelance husband
who can be around to take the kids to the dentist. And like her
husband, Blanche loves to travel. In fact, it's their mutual passion for
travel that got Krubner into the stock business in the first place.

Blanche and Ralph met at a party that they had both come to
with blind dates. Ralph was fiddling with his shiny new Rolleiflex
and it attracted Blanche like a lure attracts a salmon. They dumped
their dates and left the party together. Early in their marriage, the
Krubners resisted the status quo. In 1959 they packed their baby,
hitched a 34-foot trailer to their Rambler and headed out on a
four-year pilgrimage across the U.S. The trailer, outfitted with an 8
x 10-foot darkroom, was the mobile headquarters for Ralph's stock
business. The Krubners were not the sort of tourists who plaster
stickers on their bumper to prove they've spent a day in Yellowstone
or Mammoth Cave. Instead they'd pull into a town, hook up their

trailer and stick around long enough to record and catalogue their surroundings. Ralph shot photographs and Blanche wrote wry, precisely observed articles to send home to a local newspaper in Goshen, New York.

In 1963 they headed back east with 7,000 4 x 5 negatives and a second baby. Today a remarkable archive of Americana in the late Fifties and early Sixties is housed in Ralph and Blanche's upstairs bedroom. Prints from that trip are impeccably filed and labeled with Blanche's encyclopedic captions. "Grauman's Chinese Theater showing Jerry Lewis's *The Absent-Minded Professor.*" "A billboard on a studio backlot listing the TV series filmed there: *Leave it to Beaver* and *Alfred Hitchcock Presents.*" An Air Force missile used benignly as a sculpture in a Phoenix shopping mall, a sea of cats-eye sunglasses worn by spectators at a rodeo, 1950s-vintage motels like the one where Humbert Humbert took Lolita, with multi-colored neon signs shaped like sombreros and palm trees. These are photos so ripe with nostalgia that although they are in black and white you can see the post-war hues of pink and turquoise. "The life we led prefigured the Sixties by a decade," chirps Blanche. "We were pre-flower children."

Professionally, Krubner was 20 years ahead of his time as well. Today, clever and aggressive stock agencies have succeeded in opening up vast new markets for stock photography. It's almost always less expensive to pick up existing work than it is to assign original photography, and the stock houses are managing to convince budget-conscious clients that stock can be interesting and current. This means keeping files up to date by "assigning" stock photography to certain shooters. Agencies stockpile marketable subject matter and can deliver it before a client has to ask. Recently, a few lucky young photographers have become good enough at the stock game to give up assignment work entirely, in favor of the freedom of setting up their own shots and being their own art directors.

Although nobody knows his name in New York or Los Angeles, Krubner is a local hero at the Ocean County Camera Club, where he usually walks off with most of the ribbons, and in return, gives frequent lectures on technique. "Ralph is incredibly generous with us," says one member of this predominantly middle-aged club. "You know how some professionals hoard their secrets? Not Ralph." As far as the members are concerned, Ralph lives the life of Riley, doing for a living what they only get to do in their spare time, or after retirement. Krubner has been at the business of stock photography so long that he's a bit blasé about it. But there's no question that the travel makes up for the endless rolls of ho-hum subjects, and that Krubner is glad that he's making a living by making pictures, rather than working in an office. "I'm delighted to sort of express myself with a camera," he says. "I run into so many people who do work they don't like. I feel sorry for them."

Krubner would clearly rather "sort of" express himself with a camera than get caught up in the excesses of the ego-inflated art world. "I don't like to put anybody down," says Krubner, "but you find a lot of photography that's just too subjective. You know the examination of one's navel type of thing? Someone who is half smart develops a style which is very superficial. And that's what gets attention in the magazines and galleries. I remember a critic once said, 'After a while, I get bored with people expressing themselves, because once they're through expressing themselves, they don't express anything else.'" Ralph pauses thoughtfully. "Expressing oneself is good. I'm not against it. And I even do it myself *once* in a while."

When we interact with the medical establishment, we all need and deserve patient advocates. Please share your stories with us at our website:

http://www.weneedpatientadvocates.com/

Made in the USA
Monee, IL
04 February 2021

59658279R00111